Dr. Vagnini's

Healthy Heart Plan

*A Surgeon's Approach to Natural and Allopathic
Treatment for Cardiovascular Wellness*

Frederic J. Vagnini, MD, FACS

in cooperation with
Maria Santoro, RD

Compiled and edited by Geoffrey F. Proud

Dr. Vagnini's Healthy Heart Plan

Frederick Vagnini, MD, FACS
Maria Santoro, RD
Editor: Geoffrey F. Proud

Cover design by Paul Kreiling, PK Graphics

ISBN 1-884820-71-9
Library of Congress Catalog Card Number 2002106956

Printed in USA

Dr. Vagnini's Healthy Heart Plan is not intended as medical advice. It is written solely for informational and educational purposes. Please consult a health professional should the need for one be indicated. Because there is always some risk involved, the author and publisher are not responsible for any adverse effects or consequences resulting from the use of any of the suggestions, preparations, or methods described in this book. The publisher does not advocate the use of any particular diet or health program, but believes the information presented in this book should be available to the public.

All listed addresses, phone numbers, and fees have been reviewed and updated during production. However the data is subject to change.

Safe Goods Publishing
561 Shunpike Rd.
Sheffield, MA 01257
413-229-7935

The Author

Dr. Frederic J. Vagnini is one of the most unique physicians and health educators in the world. After graduation from St. Louis University School of Medicine (MO) in 1963, Dr. Vagnini underwent eight years of postdoctorate internship and residency at the Downstate Medical Center in Brooklyn, (NY) and Columbia Presbyterian Medical Center in New York City. Prior to entering into private practice he served in the United States Army as a Lieutenant Colonel. He is board certified in cardiothoracic surgery and surgery (FACS). He is also a fellow of the American College of Cardiology, of the American College of Nutrition, of the American College of Bariatric Medicine, and of the American Academy of Anti-Aging Medicine.

For the next twenty-five years, Dr. Vagnini practiced as a heart, lung, and blood vessel surgeon where he has operated on thousands of patients with heart and blood vessel disease. As his career continued, Dr. Vagnini became interested in health education, preventive medicine, and clinical nutrition. He has been a frequent guest speaker on radio and television regarding his experience in the heart and nutrition fields. Dr. Vagnini presently hosts a live call-in radio show on WOR in New York City. "The Heart Show" airs from 4-5 p.m. on Sundays. He previously hosted a national health show on Fox TV.

Dr. Vagnini has written hundreds of articles in the lay literature and has produced numerous scientific publications. For the last ten years he provided readers with pertinent information in his *Cardiovascular Wellness Newsletter* from which many of the chapters in this book have been extracted.

The Editor

Geoffrey F. Proud is a health care journalist who coedited the *Cardiovascular Wellness Newsletter* with Joanne Dolinar and is the founder and former editor of the New York health care monthly publication, *Hospital News*.

3

Dr. Vagnini's Cardiovascular Wellness Centers

1600 Stewart Avenue
Westbury NY 11590

944 Park Avenue
New York NY 10028

Telephone: (888) HEART-90 [432-7890]

Website: www.vagnini.com.

The Cardiovascular Wellness Centers carry a full line of vitamins and nutritional supplements. Call or write for the current catalog:
Cardiovascular Wellness Center.
Attn: Brian
1600 Stewart Ave.,
Westbury, NY 11590

also....
Listen to Dr. Vagnini, "The Prevention Doctor,"
host of THE HEART SHOW
WOR-Radio, New York, Sundays 4-5 p.m.

Foreword

Advances in scientific knowledge proceed on several fronts, optimally simultaneously. The basic researcher working in the lab doing *in vitro* and *in vivo* work provides us the crucial answers to the unique question of why an intervention reduces premature death and disability. Clinicians and nurses provide enormous benefits to patients by applying advances in treatment and diagnosis and by formulating hypotheses from their clinical experiences. The epidemiologists and statisticians formulate hypotheses from descriptive studies, correlational studies, and cross-sectional surveys, and test them in observational cohort or case-controlled studies, as well as randomized trials when needed. These studies answer the crucial and complementary question of whether an intervention reduces premature death and disability. All of these scientific disciplines provide important, relevant and complementary information contributing to a totality of evidence. At any point in time it is this totality of evidence that forms the basis for rational clinical decisions for patients, as well as policy decisions for the health of the general public.

– Dr. Charles Hennekens,
Professor of Medicine at Harvard Medical School and Director of the renowned Men's Health Study. (Newsmaker Interview, Access Excellence/The National Health Museum—www.accessexcellence.org).

Acknowledgments

As you read through this book you will surmise that it was written almost literally between patients, or at the end of a practice day after I finished dictation in my clinics at the Cardiovascular Wellness and Longevity Centers in Manhattan and on Long Island. I was assisted by my editor, Geoff Proud, who brought the topics to me—health issues that were in the news and questions that were on the mind of my patients. We sat down together in a dialogue from which came many of these news pieces. For this reason, I believe they are fresh and relevant and can contribute to the reader's personal health management program; and for this I am grateful to Geoff for his part in the book's development.

Let me also acknowledge Joanne Dolinar, who was coeditor of the *Cardiovascular Wellness Newsletter,* where many of the articles on nutrition first appeared. Joanne set up the dialogue with my nutritionist, Maria Santoro, and together they produced the section of book that offers practical tips on how to diet while keeping a healthy and inviting kitchen. My patients and my staff I also acknowledge with gratitude; they are the living context in which I pursue my profession every day. It is the interchange I maintain with them that yields not only an ever deepening understanding of the profession of healing but also renders me great personal career satisfaction.

Dr. Vagnini's Healthy Heart Plan arose from the dialogues between the editor and myself. Science has learned the cause of heart disease—specifically atherosclerosis, as the build up of fatty substances (plaques) on the walls of the coronary arteries, much of which we introduce through our diets. Experts know how to prevent plaque buildup with the application of TLC (therapeutic life changes), chiefly proper diet and exercise. To assist in this process, we've developed magnificent drugs, marvelous surgeries, and many natural supplements. I challenge you to prove that heart disease can be cured in our lifetime by absorbing the information you find in this book and taking your heart health into your own hands.

-Frederic Vagnini MD, FACS
Westbury and Manhattan, NY

Introduction

The professional career of Dr. Fred Vagnini has been a dedicated path toward improving the health of those who have come to him, and of reaching out to others with the wisdom gained from his study, experience, and the generosity of his spirit. During his twenty-five years as a cardiovascular surgeon, he not only repaired his patients' hearts with skilled hands but also assured them with his counsel. Transitioning to preventive practice, he has been a leader for over a decade in the use of advanced contemporary medical science for the diagnosis and treatment of many ailments relating to cardiovascular disease—heart attack, stroke, hypertension, diabetes, and embraces the principles of antiaging medicine.

In addition to his clinical practice in the Cardiovascular Wellness and Longevity Centers on Long Island and on Park Avenue in New York City, he has contributed as a popular health educator through writings in his newsletter and professional journals, and in his radio call-in program on WOR 710, New York City, *The Heart Show.*

This book is an extension of his role as a health educator. It has always been a tenet of Dr. Vagnini's that knowledge is an essential component of good health. Today, more than ever, with the rapid progress being made in the development of health promoting drugs and in the design of life-saving medical instruments, health care consumers must be kept abreast of the benefits that are available to them. The materials collected in this book are drawn from the most recent findings and reports outlined in medical literature. They have been selected, interpreted, and commented on by Dr. Vagnini with the intention of making them of practical use to his readers.

Some of the pieces in the book have been circulated to his patients in the *Cardiovascular Wellness Newsletter.* Others were written especially for this publication and represent the health news of the day. Altogether they reflect Dr. Vagnini's deep professional interest in the myriad aspects of modern health care and medical science: new and powerful drugs, surgical techniques, nutritional supplements, and prevention principles. The book aligns with the current emphasis on the root metabolic causes of cardiovascular diseases and includes a section on insulin resistance. But the balance is general health news and information valuable for all health care consumers, presented in a journalistic style for easy understanding and laid out for easy selection.

In the sign-off of his radio show Dr. Vagnini reminds his audience: "Heart attacks and strokes can be prevented; your health is in your own hands." Readers who take his advice to heart (no pun intended) may find subjects that particularly pertain to them or their friends and family. They may also discover issues they are curious about, having heard of them in the popular media.

When he is not at his desk dictating his commentary on these subjects to this editor, Dr. Vagnini is active in his Centers. These facilities include the most sophisticated equipment for diagnostics, such as stress tests, sonographic vascular imaging, and as a diet and nutritional department directed by Maria Santoro, who has contributed the diet advice and nutritional comment.

May *Dr. Vagnini's Healthy Heart Plan* make you healthier.

-Geoffrey F. Proud, Editor

Table of Contents

Prologue

Much of the health education information provided in this book is based on findings of scientific studies reported in popular and professional publications. As there are many references to scientific studies in the articles that follow, it is of value to consider the methodologies by which medical findings are arrived at.

Statistical studies are of two kinds: observational and interventional. The former is a study in which peoples' behavior and lifestyle is analyzed and quantified in order to establish important facts. A prime example is the research that determined the connection between lung cancer and smoking. This kind of research is called *epidemiological research*. It counts the number of cases gathered from findings and analyzes huge databases in order to draw conclusions. The famous Framingham Heart Study[1], which determined the risk factors for heart disease is another example. In this study, researchers recruited 5209 men and women from the town of Framingham, Massachusetts, and collected data through extensive physical examinations and lifestyle interviews over a period of 50 years.

Interventional research is typically the *double-blind clinical trial*. In this type of study, researchers set up two groups of subjects and compare the effects of treatments. "Double-blind" means that neither the subjects nor the researchers know which group has received the test treatment, and which the placebo, an inactive substance. This research is usually done with smaller groups of subjects that can be controlled by the researchers. The larger the group, the more stable will be the statistical findings. For this reason, it is important to know how many subjects were involved in the study in order to judge the reliability of the reported results. Knowing the source of the research report is also important. As good as it is to have pharmaceutical companies underwrite the cost of research, the risk is that the reports will be biased. Nevertheless, there is always valuable information to be found in these reports—even if they are slanted. It only requires that the reader be discriminating.

Persons who follow the reports of medical research can become confused when one report appears to contradict another. But consistency

---

[1] The Framingham Heart Study, a major tracking study since 1948 continues to produce valuable research data for heart disease.
www.nhlbi.nih.gov/about/framingham/index.html.

of evidence is important. A discerning inquirer will conclude that if a large of number of studies all show the same thing and one study seems to contradict it, it is unlikely that 20 studies are wrong and this one is right. That defies logic. Our health education knowledge base does not shift back and forth as more findings of science are added to it. It is cumulative, and as it grows our discernment is more acute and our ability to convert it into good health practice becomes surer. It takes time to investigate and interpret all the factors that influence our health. Scientists pursue questions over and over again. Not every scientific "breakthrough" is the final answer. The quest goes on. As you read with informed critical judgment, you will become more adept at extracting medical information that is beneficial to your personal health.

Chapter One
Prevention is Prime

On my desk, turned outward for my patients to see, is a plaque inscribed with the words "The Prevention Doctor." It is a token of appreciation given to me by friends. After listening to me on the radio for an hour every week for many years, it was their assessment that the theme of my practice is prevention. I graciously accept the title if it will impress on my audience the primacy of prevention. My weekly radio call-in show has been a major feature of my health education efforts. It gives me an opportunity to review for the audience the current news in health care, especially those reports that pertain to cardiovascular wellness and offer more possibilities for prevention of disease. Much of this you will be reading as your get further into this book. The radio show is also a source of feedback from the public, telling me how they are coping with their health problems.

Over many years of this activity, I have been able to hone to a precise plan what I call the "Ten Steps to a Healthy Heart." My mantra declares that most heart attacks and strokes can be prevented. What a hopeful notion that is when you consider that heart attacks and strokes are the number one and number three killers of Americans.

While the most spectacular happenings in health care may be scientific breakthrough therapies and procedures, health care's most important aspect is truly prevention. When I speak to an audience of health care consumers, the first thing I do is lay down my principles for the prevention of heart attack and stroke. The discussion of these ten steps will help you understand many notions and themes that you will find as you read further. But, of course, once you study them you will want to put these principles into practice.

Ten Steps to a Healthy Heart

1. *Take advantage of health education programs.* Pay attention to experts wherever you may find them—on radio, in your reading, or on the Internet. In health education books like the one you are presently

15

reading, I try to present the latest in research and developments in heart disease. I make this information practical in the light of my experience of treating thousands of patients for heart and circulation problems in my Wellness and Longevity Centers in Manhattan and Westbury, New York.

2. ***Research your family history.*** A brand new study indicates that if there is a family history of cardiovascular disease, even if you are asymptomatic, you have a 50 percent chance of having a cardiovascular problem. This study was based on PET scanning, (a high-tech nuclear imaging system for early detection of heart disease and preventing its further development). Prevention is possible and these methods are extremely important in producing favorable results. Often someone will come into my office and say, "I thought I should see you, Doc, because I'm 49½ and my father had a heart attack at age 50." I say, "Fine, but don't you think you're cutting it close? You should have been here much sooner." I have always said that most heart attacks and strokes can be prevented. Persons who have a history of premature heart disease in their family should be treated early and just as aggressively as if they have heart disease. The same preventive approach goes for stroke and diabetes. Diabetes doubles a person's likelihood of having a heart attack.

3. ***Start your preventive practices early.*** A heart attack or stroke does not just happen the day you go into the hospital for emergency treatment or for a balloon angioplasty or bypass surgery. It begins many years earlier. Research using intravascular ultrasound scanning at the Cleveland Clinic, showed that one out of six teenagers have the beginnings of heart disease. In the Bogaloosa Heart Study,[2] children as young as seven were found to have early atherosclerosis. The famous Korean War Heart Study[3] showed that 20-year-old soldiers had significant coronary disease. The lesson from these

---

[2] The Bogalusa Heart Study (since 1972 out of Louisiana State University Medical Center) is the longest and most detailed study of children in the world. The focus is on understanding the early natural history of coronary artery disease and essential hypertension. It is the only major program studying a well-defined, biracial (black-white) population of children in a total semi-rural community. The community represents the southeastern United States. www.som.tulane.edu/cardiohealth/bog.htm.

[3] Heart Risk Factor Lab. During the Korean War, doctors were surprised to find that the hearts of many young men killed in battle had already begun to develop coronary artery disease. Search the Internet for "Korean War Heart Disease."

findings is, "Don't wait for a heart attack to strike." This is a preventable disease.

4. ***Look for the disease before symptoms occur.*** Atherosclerosis is a slow process. It starts in youth and is influenced by secondary and multiple risk factors. Waiting until you have chest pains is not the time to be examined. The time to get a preventive cardiac workup is when you are in your 40s. In addition to listening to heart rhythms and observing your pulse, a good preventive workup includes various blood tests to measure lipid levels (cholesterol), an EKG, and in some cases, vascular ultrasound imagining. If there are indications, a stress test may be in order. I call this "The Healthy Heart Program" at my centers. Testing before symptoms occur can be a problem with HMO insurers. They tend to deny referrals if there are no symptoms, sometimes even for symptoms they consider minor. This can be especially risky for women, because women do not experience the same kind of symptoms of heart disease men experience. Today, one of the most sophisticated methods for diagnosing coronary disease is coronary CT scanning. This technology detects calcifications in the coronary arteries, which we know are an early warning sign for disease.

5. ***Reduce risk factors.*** This is the key to your personal healthy heart plan. We know what the risk factors are: smoking, hypertension, high cholesterol and other lipid levels, excess weight. All you really have to do is know what risk factors you might have, get checked, and then take the steps to get the numbers in line. An elevated homocysteine level is now also recognized as one of the independent risk factors for heart disease. It should be measured in every blood test you have. And as I have been teaching for years, it can be managed not with prescription drugs but with nutritional supplements— folic acid taken with vitamin B6 and B12. Since we know the risk factors for heart disease, and since we also know how to deal with them, we are moving toward curing heart disease. It is just up to each individual to follow these steps.

6. ***Focus on antioxidants.*** The scientific community now believes that most atherosclerosis is due to oxidized LDL (low density lipid cholesterol), which sets off the production of free radicals, which in turn damage cells lining the blood vessels. The nutritional substances

17

that are known to counter free radical activity are vitamins E and C, and beta-carotene. Vitamin C is plentiful in most diets in citrus fruits and vegetables. Vegetables, seed oils, eggs, and liver are good sources of vitamin E. (For cardiovascular protection, diet may not supply enough vitamin E and it should be taken in supplements.) Beta-carotene is found in yellow vegetables, including carrots. Our bodies also naturally produce antioxidant compounds such as lipoic acid, CoEnzyme Q10, and glutathione. However, recent research findings have shown that human production of these naturally produced antioxidants is insufficient for optimal defense against free radical damage; therefore supplemental nutrients may be necessary. Antioxidant therapy is important for blood vessel wall function and for lowering LDL. Scientific researchers are now showing that antioxidants are even beneficial in preventing Alzheimer's and Parkinson's diseases.

7. *Control your emotions and stress.* I've always said three things cause a heart attack: shoveling snow, a fight with your wife, or having the IRS after you. Emotions, hostility, and anger have all been associated with heart attacks. We all have problems to deal with; that is why it is so important to have your body in good shape. If you are physically healthy, you are in a position to fight off these high stress situations, and will have one less thing to worry about.

8. *Maintain a healthy weight.* Obesity is an epidemic in this country. It is associated with every health problem we have been talking about: hypertension, heart disease, stroke, and early death. You should maintain a weight of *metabolic fitness*—which means a weight at which your blood pressure is OK, your insulin levels are OK, your cholesterol and triglycerides are under control, you feel good, and can live an active life. That's metabolic fitness. Activity is an important factor too; because excessive weight will slow you down and make you feel tired all the time.

    If you need to lose weight there are many programs that will help you. The diet I outline in this book is an *insulin regulating diet* that has proven to be very successful. As people get older, they naturally put on weight. It is only a problem if it indicates some other health trouble. I find that among many of the women who come into my office their weight problem is associated with high blood pressure, diabetes, or arthritis.

9. *Learn about the "cholesterol controversy."* High levels of cholesterol in the blood are associated with greater numbers of heart attacks. In May 2001, the National Cholesterol Education Program issued new and stricter guidelines to follow: 200 is the desirable level for total cholesterol, 100 for LDL cholesterol. I firmly support and recommend these because I believe in the importance of maintaining a lower cholesterol level, and this can be done in many cases by natural means. The majority of lipid problems can be treated by natural therapies. The key nutrients are magnesium, chromium, niacin, panathene, carnathene, essential oils, and the very powerful red yeast rice, which is similar in its effect to the drugs they give for lowering cholesterol.

    I am not opposed to using drugs for lowering cholesterol if the level is extremely high and cannot be lowered by natural means. When a young man comes into my office with a moderate cholesterol level of 230, I don't recommend that he be put on statin drugs for the rest of his life. Natural therapies will often do the trick. There is really no cholesterol controversy; that notion arose at a time when they thought 300 was a desirable level. Much more is now known about cholesterol. Yes, people may suffer a heart attack even with low cholesterol levels of around 200, but other factors, such as high triglycerides and very low HDL cholesterol, also add to the risk.

10. *Learn about diabetes, impaired glucose tolerance, and insulin resistance.* Currently there is an epidemic of insulin resistance, and the national health experts have recognized this. (See Chapter Nine.) It is described sometimes as "Syndrome X," which is a metabolic syndrome characterized by central abdominal obesity (fat stomach), high triglycerides and high cholesterol, impaired glucose tolerance, and high blood pressure. This syndrome is often associated as well with high uric acid, and now we are finding, in men with sexual dysfunction and low levels of testosterone. If you have a weight problem and you're tired all the time, there is a very good chance you are a diabetic or prediabetic—in spite of your fasting blood sugar. People who have no suspicion that they are diabetic come to my centers every week. After a glucose test, we find that they are diabetic or prediabetic.

Your Cholesterol Levels

Aggressive cholesterol management will not only stop the progression of coronary artery disease, it can actually reverse it. People may think of cholesterol management as the lowering of the total cholesterol level, but it is important to look at each element of your lipid profile individually. Your doctor can provide you with your cholesterol profile, and you should be aware of what the numbers mean. The cholesterol profile consists of total cholesterol, high-density lipid (HDL) cholesterol, low-density lipid (LDL) cholesterol, triglycerides, and the ratio of HDL to total cholesterol and the ratio of LDL (bad) to HDL (good). Very recently the National Cholesterol Education Program (NCEP) has stressed the importance of lowering the measure of LDL to below 100 for maximum safety (see the new cholesterol guidelines in this chapter). For prevention of heart disease and its symptoms and effects, every effort should be made to lower one's LDL to that standard, if not by diet restrictions, then by using drugs.

No drugs have been targeted at HDL, the good cholesterol, although it is also important to keep it in line. Researchers have estimated that for every 1% increase in HDL cholesterol you will decrease your chances of getting coronary artery disease by 3-4%. The desirable HDL level is above 45. Although a high total cholesterol level or a high LDL (bad) cholesterol level significantly increases your risk for heart disease, if it is accompanied by a high HDL cholesterol level, the risk can be substantially lowered.

On the other hand, many people who have heart attacks have normal total cholesterol, but their HDL cholesterol level is low—below 40. The NCEP recommends that even people with normal total cholesterol levels should have their HDL cholesterol levels checked. Here are some ways to raise your HDL level:

- Exercise – Exercise is a very effective way to raise HDL levels. Thirty minutes of exercise three to four times a week is needed to make a difference. Those who exercise will probably experience an increase in HDL levels after six to eight weeks.
- Lose weight – HDL levels rise as weight decreases. On the basis of HDL levels alone, inactive men can expect to have coronary heart disease at three times the rate of athletic men.
- Use monounsaturated oils – Olive, peanut, and canola oils and oils from most nuts and seeds are monounsaturated and will help raise HDL levels. Hydrogenated oil, which is found in margarine and used

extensively in processed foods and for deep-frying in fast food restaurants, is to be avoided.

- <u>Drink alcohol moderately</u> – Alcohol in moderation decreases the risk of heart attack because it raises the HDL level. Keep in mind that although moderate consumption protects the heart, heavy alcohol consumption is a leading cause of death.
- <u>Take niacin and chromium</u> – Immediate release niacin will provide a significant increase in HDL cholesterol, and it has fewer serious side effects than the sustained-release variety. Niacin, although not a drug, should only be taken under a physician's direction. Chromium picolinate taken daily raises HDL levels while reducing total cholesterol. Like niacin, it should only be taken on the advice of a physician.
- <u>Quit smoking</u> – Smoking lowers the HDL levels for both smokers and their children. Most of the damage done by cigarettes is a result of the smoke interfering with the HDL processes in the body. People who exercise regularly but smoke will not experience a rise in HDL level.
- <u>Women should consider some form of hormone therapy</u> – Women experience a drop in HDL level after menopause, but hormone therapy may effectively counteract the decrease and raise HDL levels.

At this time, drug therapy is not recommended to treat low HDL in patients unless it is in conjunction with drug therapy to lower LDL or total cholesterol levels. In fact, the NHLBI recommends delaying the use of any cholesterol lowering medications as long possible, especially for younger men and women. Making lifestyle changes to lower LDL, and raise HDL cholesterol levels may mean that you won't ever find it necessary to take drugs for cholesterol management.

The New Cholesterol Guidelines

The publication in May 3, 2001 of the report of the National Cholesterol Education Program's Adult Treatment Panel[4] is good news for America's health. It establishes a stricter set of guidelines for the diagnosis and treatment of heart disease, the country's number one killer, and it puts behind us any controversy about the importance of blood lipid management in the prevention of heart attacks and strokes. Whereas the

---

[4] National Institutes of Health (NIH), *National Cholesterol Education Program,* www.nihbi.nih.gov/guidelines/cholesterol.

national health monitoring and research agencies had once accepted a level for LDL (low density lipid) cholesterol of below 130 as "desirable," they now call for a level of below 100 as "optimal" — a reassessment of 30 or more points! They also emphasize that the LDL level is the key factor in assessing risk for heart disease in a lipoprotein profile, rather than total cholesterol. These guidelines are the first major update from NCEP in nearly a decade. The new guideline chart looks like this:

Low Density Lipid (LDL) Cholesterol
BELOW 100	OPTIMAL
100-129	Near to Above Optimal
130-159	Borderline High
160-189	High
Above 190	Very High

High Density Lipid (HDL) Cholesterol
Below 40	Low
Above 60	High

Total Cholesterol
Below 200	Desirable
200-239	Borderline High
Above 240	High

According to the press statement released by the National Cholesterol Education Program of the National Institutes of Health, the new guidelines present very specific recommendations and precise statistical ranges for the treatment of patients whose risk for heart disease is identified in their lipid profile, starting with the LDL level. Three categories are established for patients identified with elevated LDL.

1. For patients with known atherosclerosis (coronary heart disease), LDL should be reduced to below 100 with TLC (Therapeutic Lifestyle Changes). But if LDL is above 130, then drug therapy should be considered.

2. For patients with no evidence of heart disease but with two or more risk factors—such as smoking, family history, diabetes, age over 50, or low HDL—then LDL should be in the near-optimal

22

range, below 130, achieved by TLC. Consider drugs to reduce the 10-year risk of disease to under 20 percent.

3. For patients with elevated LDL, but with one or less additional risk factors, who have a 10-year risk of heart disease lower than 10 percent, their LDL should be no greater than 159, the borderline high level.

Other key measurements in the NCEP guidelines are the HDL and triglyceride levels. HDL below 40 is considered a risk factor for heart disease. It had formerly been below 35. Triglycerides are to be monitored in relation to LDL levels and treatment is recommended for triglyceride levels at 200 or above. Below 150 is considered the normal range for triglycerides.

Therapeutic Lifestyle Changes (TLC) are precisely defined by the Panel: a daily diet with saturated fat making up less than 7 percent of caloric intake, less that 200 mg of cholesterol, increased voluble fiber and vegetables, weight management, and increased physical activity. The report also identifies a cluster of heart disease risk factors, which it calls "the metabolic syndrome." For years specialists in the field of preventive medicine have know this as "*Syndrome X.*" This syndrome includes too much abdominal fat (waist measurement over 40 inches), hypertension, high triglycerides, and low HDL. It is indicative of insulin resistance, a disorder of the insulin function in the body's metabolism, and the underlying cause of Type 2 diabetes. It is treated by intense TLC. (Insulin resistance is discussed at length in a later section of this book.)

According to the press statement released by the National Institutes of Health, of which the National Cholesterol Education Program is a function, the new guidelines will increase the number of Americans being treated for high cholesterol. They are expected to increase the number of persons who are prescribed a cholesterol-lowering drug from about 13 million to about 35 million—an increase of over 175 percent. They will also increase the number of those on dietary treatment from about 52 million to about 65 million. NCEP is decisively addressing the problem of too many Americans at high risk for heart attacks and strokes whose risk goes undetected and untreated. For too many Americans a heart attack is the first symptom that indicates they have heart disease. Experts believe also that the foundation for heart disease is often laid in adolescence and early adulthood. An early recognition of risk factors and aggressive treatment can result in long-term prevention of the life-threatening effects of the disease.

Exercise Can Keep You Young

The blood vessels of older athletes behave like those of people half their age, says a new study out of Italy reported in *Circulation,* the journal of the American Heart Association.[5] Dr. Taddei and his researchers studied sedentary individuals versus athletes, young and old. The athletes were long-distance runners, cyclists and triathletes, who combined running, cycling, and swimming. Both groups of young people, the sedentary and the athletes, averaged 27 years of age. The average ages for the older groups were 63 for the sedentary and 65 for the athletes. The study found that the older athletes' blood vessels functioned as well as those of the participants in either of the two younger groups. "This study demonstrates that regular physical activity can protect aging blood vessels," says the study's lead author, Stefano Taddei M.D., an associate professor of internal medicine at the University of Pisa in Italy. "Long-term exercise protects the inner lining of the blood vessels from age-related changes and makes them behave more like those of a younger person."

It may not take a triathlon to reap benefits. A study by the Honolulu Heart Program published in *Circulation* last year showed that regularly walking more than 1.5 miles a day reduced heart disease risk in older individuals.[6] You do not need to be an athlete to get these beneficial effects from exercise. As I have often insisted, aerobic activity five days a week—rather than intensive training—might just do the trick. Blood vessels need to be able to expand in order to accommodate increases in blood flow. A protective layer of cells, called the endothelium, produces a substance called nitric oxide that helps the vessels dilate when the heart needs more blood. Nitric oxide also protects the vessel walls from developing atherosclerosis (the buildup of fatty substances that thicken the arteries and block blood flow) and thrombosis (the formation of blood clots that can block small or narrowed vessels and cause heart attacks)

---

[5] Taddei, Stefano, et al., *Physical Activity Prevents Age-Related Impairment in Nitric Oxide Availability in Elderly Athletes,* Circulation vol. 101 (2000), http.//circ.ahajournals.org/search.dtl.

[6] Hakim, A.A., et al., *Effects of walking on coronary heart disease in elderly men: the Honolulu Heart Program.* Circulation, vol. 100 (1999), http.//circ.ahajournals.org/search.dtl.

according to Dr. Stefano Taddai. Aging can cause alterations in the endothelium, he says, making older individuals more prone to atherosclerosis and thrombosis.

Previous studies have linked aging to problems in endothelium responsiveness and have shown that exercise can make the endothelium dilate more efficiently, even for patients with chronic heart failure. In the Italian study, Dr. Taddei's team looked at 12 young and 12 older sedentary subjects and compared them to 11 young athletes and 14 older athletes. The researchers gave the study subjects a substance called *acetyicholine*, which causes the blood vessels to dilate if the endothelium is producing nitric oxide properly. The young subjects, whether sedentary or active, had similar strong responses to acetyicholine, and their vessels dilated. Among the older participants, athletes showed greater blood vessel dilation than the sedentary group.

Another age-related change in the endothelium as we age is increased free radicals in the blood. Free radicals are highly unstable reactive oxygen molecules that circulate in the blood and damage tissues. These reactive molecules play a major role in the formation of artery-blocking fatty buildup when they come in contact with LDL cholesterol, the "bad" cholesterol. Scientists believe that exercise and certain vitamins have antioxidant effects by blocking free radicals. The researchers found in this study that older athletes had lower blood levels of free radicals similar to the younger study subjects. However, the older sedentary individuals had high levels of free radicals and their blood vessels showed dilation only when the researchers administered high doses of the antioxidant, vitamin C.

Lifestyle Physical Activity

Don't get enough exercise? No time to go to the fitness center? Find working out too hard and no fun? Not to worry; we have learned in studies over the past decade that even if you cannot undertake a structured physical fitness program, the amount of exercise necessary to achieve health benefits could be obtained in the routine of your daily life.[7] Researchers now say that the amount of exercise necessary for health benefits is considerably less than the amount needed to become physically fit. Twenty years ago, the general belief was that if a person did not exercise

---

[7] *Simple Lifestyle Changes Boost Physical Activity/Cardiovascular Health,* WEBMD—http://my.webmd.com/content/article/1680/50398.

within a given heart rate range or exercise intensity, the benefits of the program would be minimal. It's not surprising that most people could not adopt intensive exercise programs and that 60 percent of Americans have remained sedentary. The good news is that even low to moderate intensity physical activity, typical of everyday life, has favorable effects on cardiometabolic health. These benefits include improved glucose homeostasis, blood lipid-lipoprotein levels, abdominal fat distribution, and blood pressure—even though they may not necessarily result in substantial gains in physical fitness and weight loss.

The principle however, remains as always—the most effective method for long-term weight loss maintenance is a combination of caloric restriction achieved by dietary restriction and increased caloric expenditure through an exercise program. That this principle may be upheld through "lifestyle physical activity" is what experts now contend. Lifestyle physical activity is defined as the daily accumulation of at least 30 minutes of self-selected activities, which includes all leisure, occupational, or household activities that are at least moderate in their intensity and could be planned or unplanned activities that are part of everyday life. The advantage of this program is that it is more likely to motivate people who are otherwise sedentary, because these activities are easily within the realm of their daily lives. In practice, lifestyle physical activity is recommended on a daily or near daily basis. They could take anywhere from 10 to 60 minutes in two or three sessions a day. Being of moderate intensity means that the heart rate will be half or less of what might be reached on a graded exercise stress test. Typical of everyday life might be three 10-minute walks per day, using the stairs rather than the elevator at work, a brief workout with hand weights and stretching exercises.

Also important to make lifestyle physical activity work is the counsel of the physician. In the massive Behavioral Risk Factor Surveillance System[8] survey recently conducted among over 20,000 adult subjects in seven states, researchers established that physicians counseled 40 percent of the respondents on preventive measures, such as exercise and a healthier diet, to avoid coronary heart disease. Those who receive advice from their physicians are more likely to adjust their lifestyle than those not counseled. Studies like this are ongoing and have a twofold objective; to lay a statistical foundation in clinical practice for defining the necessary behavior for maintaining good cardiovascular health, and to identify the role of both the patient and the physician in reaching that goal.

---

[8] Centers for Disease Control (CDC), www.cdc.gov/nccdphp/brfss.

Need a Daily Reminder?

The American Heart Association has initiated a program called "One of a Kind," in which Internet respondents may register and receive an almost daily reminder to behave in a heart-healthy manner.[9] The registration form asks for personal information relating to one's risks of cardiovascular problems such as age, physical statistics, any past history of heart problems, and so forth. Privacy is assured. This is to enable AHA to "personalize" a daily health advisory for you. For example, on March 17 the message adopted a St. Patrick's Day theme—"Instead of only wearing green, eat some leafy green vegetables; they're a great source of fiber and fiber is an important component to a healthy eating plan." The advice continued on with more information about fiber in the diet, "If you eat it regularly, soluble fiber can help lower your blood cholesterol level." Soluble fiber is found in oat bran, oatmeal, peas, beans, and citrus foods. Insoluble fiber is found in leafy green vegetables, whole wheat breads and cereals, cabbage, beats, carrots, Brussels sprouts, turnips, and cauliflower. The AHA web site reminder then goes on to offer a St. Patrick's Day recipe, Quick Green Bean Casserole. In a microwave, it takes only five minutes and, according to the information supplied, would include 0 g of saturated fat, only 2 mg of cholesterol, and 55 calories per serving. Sign up at www.onelife.americanheart.org. It's free!

No Letup in Stroke Prevention

In the last decade, the mortality rate from stroke has declined by about one-third. Can we assume that in another ten years the rate will drop by a third again, and by ten years after that we will have eliminated stroke altogether? Sorry, it doesn't work that way. Our vigilance over cardiovascular disease has to be constant; and health education, which is the essence of prevention, must continue as each new generation comes along.

About 145,000 persons die as a result of stroke every year. It is the leading killer after heart attack and all forms of cancer combined. We've learned that lifestyle changes, among other preventive steps, will continue to lower the mortality rate of stroke. Some of the risk factors for stroke cannot be controlled, while others can. Stroke is strongly related to age: 72 percent of its victims are over 65; men have a 19 percent higher rate of

---

[9] American Heart Association (AHA), www.onelife.americanheart.org.

stroke than women. African-American men have a death rate from stroke of 57.9 per 100,000 persons versus 46.6 per 100,000 for white men. If you have a family history of stroke, you are much more likely to suffer from one than someone who does not.[10]

Diabetics are at high risk for stroke, particularly if they also have high blood pressure. If you've had a prior stroke or a transient alchemic attack (TIA), you are at greater risk than someone who has not. Nonetheless, there is quite a lot you can do to prevent stroke. The most important step to take is to take control of lowering your blood pressure. Your risk of stroke increases as your blood pressure rises. Many people can control blood pressure by losing weight and learning to eat properly, (see the chapter in this book on Natural Therapies to Lower Your Blood Pressure). If natural therapies fail, drugs to control blood pressure are available. The second most important thing you can do is stop smoking. It is hard to believe that some people still have not gotten that message; in fact, some 50 million Americans still smoke. It is also important to avoid passive smoke. Experts estimate that about 50,000 people each year die from exposure to other people's tobacco smoke.

An increase in red blood cell count is a risk for stroke. If you suspect you are in a risk category for stroke, have your red blood count checked. If it is high, it can be treated with blood thinners. Fibrinogen is a substance produced by the body to regulate the clotting of blood. A high fibrinogen level is an independent factor for stroke. The desirable level of fibrinogen is between 200 and 400mg daily. Ask your physician to determine your fibrinogen level. Fish oils will lower fibrinogen. Smokers tend to have high fibrinogen levels, but if they stop smoking, their levels will go down.

A transient ischemic attack (TIA), which is a "mini-stroke," precedes about 10 percent of strokes. Know the symptoms of a TIA and get immediate medical attention if you have one. The symptoms resemble an actual stroke, except that they are milder: temporary loss of feeling or weakness on one side of the body; temporary loss of vision, especially in one eye only or double vision; temporary loss of speech or difficulty in speaking; dizziness; and sudden severe headache. In a TIA, these symptoms last only a short time—probably less than five minutes.

Heart disease also doubles the risk of stroke. Therefore know the risk of factors for heart disease: high cholesterol levels, obesity, and lack of exercise; these are secondary risk factors for stroke. Strokes are most

---

[10] Updated stroke statistics are found at www.americanheart.org.

likely to occur in either very hot or very cold weather. They strike the poor more often than the affluent. People in the southeastern United States are most likely to have strokes (stroke belt). It is important to remember that while some of these risk factors can't be eliminated, others can be modified with your physician's help; and still others can be greatly reduced by your own vigilance.

Prevention Notes: Stroke and Alzheimer's

A *Time* magazine story discussed research on the factors that influence the onset and progression of Alzheimer's disease (AD).[11] Four million Americans are believed to suffer from AD. Statistics indicate that on average 10 percent of people over 65 come down with Alzheimer's and that percentage rises to 50 percent by age 85. The *Time* story told of a researcher who was able to identify mental and emotional factors associated with Alzheimer's disease in a decade-long study of a convent of religions nuns in Minnesota, (i.e. "The Nuns Study.") Confirmation of a diagnosis of AD requires an autopsy in which brain cells are examined for integrity. Those found to be tangled and damaged by plaques are evident in persons whose mental capacity had severely deteriorated late in life. The researchers found that among nuns with physical evidence of Alzheimer's in the brain, those who also had evidence of strokes almost inevitably showed outwards symptoms of dementia. The study reported in *Time* is said to be among the first "to look at the cardiovascular component of Alzheimer's disease."

From this point, it is fair to conclude that therapies which might prevent strokes, will also protect against Alzheimer's: avoid tobacco, get regular exercise, and eat a cardiovascular healthy diet. Earlier research on Alzheimer's disease has found that its victims have low concentrates of folic acid in their blood. Folic acid has been effective in treating dangerously high levels of homocysteine, one of the risk factors for heart disease. Going further in finding preventive therapies to counter AD, researchers have been able to establish that the statin drugs used to manage cholesterol levels in the blood also are likely to protect against Alzheimer's disease. The statins inhibit the production of substances that compose the plaques commonly found in Alzheimer's diseased brain cells. It is encouraging to know that if you have been attentive to your regimen for cardiovascular

---

[11] Belluck, Pam, "Nun's Offer Clues to Alzheimers and Aging," *Time Magazine*, May 8, 2002.

health with proper diet and exercise, have included vitamin supplements like folic acid (B complex), and have been compliant in taking your cholesterol lowering drugs if they are prescribed, you will realize the added bonus of protecting yourself against Alzheimer's disease.

Chapter Two
Heart Health and Drugs

Statins: A Need for Information

In August 2001, the *New York Times,* as well as other media, reported the recall from the marketplace of the anti-lipid drug *Baycol.* Baycol is produced by Bayer (famous for its aspirin). It was on the market for about four years, and had been extremely profitable for the pharmaceutical company. The media reports discussed Baycol as one of the family of statin drugs, universally prescribed for lowering cholesterol and reducing the risk of cardiovascular diseases. Underlying this news were negative implications for all statin drugs. Are statins a problem? Baycol was said to have been implicated in the death of patients. Its muscle deterioration effect led to complications with the kidneys. Some of the patients affected were also taking another anti-lipid drug, a firbrate, called *gemfibrozil* (contrary to packaging instructions).

There are five very popular statin drugs prescribed for patients with serious and resistant cholesterol problems. They have the brand names Lipitor, Lescol, Mevacor, Pravachol, and Zocor. They are in a class of drugs also known as *HMG-CoA reductase inhibitors.* That is, they work by blocking an enzyme that is needed by the body to make cholesterol. Thus, less cholesterol is made. Although there once was a controversy over the value of lowering cholesterol levels in preventing cardiovascular disease, the effectiveness of the statin drugs to accomplish this is firmly established. Researchers writing in the *Journal of the American Medical Association*[12] analyzed data from randomized clinical trials conducted between 1985 and 1996 and involving 26, 000 persons. They concluded that the statins were not only effective in reducing the incidence of cardiovascular disease and death, but they in no way increased risk of death and disease from other than cardiovascular problems. All of the statin drugs

---

[12] LaRosa, John C., et al. *Effect of Statins on Risk of Coronary Diseases: A Meta-analysis of Randomized Controlled Trials.* Journal of the American Medical Association (JAMA), Vol. 282, December 22, 1999.

mentioned above were tested in one or the other of the trials over a period of about 40 months. Overall the participants in the trials benefited by a near 30 percent reduced risk of cardiovascular diseases and over 20 percent reduced risk of death from cardiovascular disease.

Experts who commented on these analyses have confirmed that "treatment with statins to reduce cholesterol significantly reduces death due to heart disease, and that previous concerns about cholesterol reduction being safe are not founded with this class of statin drugs [as] there were no safety issues raised in these trials with over 29,000 patients."

This does not mean, however, that there are no precautions to be observed in the use of statins. The first principal is to observe the instruction issued by the manufacturer and printed out with each prescription. All statin drugs are rigorously tested in hundreds of trials before they are put on the market. Nonetheless, there is always the danger of drugs being used in combinations by a patient. For this reason, patients must advise their physician of all the drugs they are taking before they begin a regimen of statins. In the case of Baycol, taking it at the same time with *gemfibrozil* proved to be dangerous. The blood-thinning drug Coumadin is also known to cause dangerous interactions with statins.

It is important to begin a regimen of statins gradually, taking lower dosages in the beginning and increasing the dosage step by step as the drug's effectiveness in lowering cholesterol is monitored. This allows the body to adjust to the medications and side effects are avoided. Some of those side effects, though rare, are upset stomach, gas, constipation, and cramps. Statins are also known to affect muscles, causing soreness and weakness. Such occurrences should be reported to the prescribing physician and the drug should be discontinued. In general, however, the disadvantages of taking statins are minor and are far outweighed by the advantages they may afford persons with risk of cardiovascular disease.

It is recommended that statins be taken in a pill once a day, preferably in the evening, because cholesterol is released in the body during the night. Keep the medication dosage even and do not double up if you miss a day. The results of statin therapy will usually show up in several weeks, at which time blood test measurements of LDL levels should be taken together with liver functions tests to be certain no adverse side effects are occurring.

If a patient is unable to tolerate statins, there are alternatives. Niacin, an over-the-counter food supplement lowers lipids and raises HDL. It is available in forms that make it easily tolerable and does not require a prescription, and yet it should be taken with the advice and counsel of a physician. Fibrates, like those sold under the brand names Lopid and Tricor, have also proven effective in regulating blood cholesterol. Always, dietary discipline and a regular exercise program are the first order of therapy for maintaining a healthy cardiovascular system—including good cholesterol levels. Statins or other drug alternatives are only recommended when diet and exercise can't get the job done.

Statins were developed primarily to treat diseases characterized by lipid disorders, but in subsequent trials have been found to be beneficial for other health problems. Diabetics will benefit from statin therapy because they are in the risk category for cardiovascular disease. Health experts now believe that persons whose cholesterol levels may not be high, but who have other risk factors for heart disease and stroke, would do well to use statin drugs. Recently, a national health authority, the National Cholesterol Education Program, has amplified its recommendation for cholesterol management.[13] By calling for an LDL (low density lipid) cholesterol level of 100 or below for "optimal" heart health, the number of persons for whom statins may be recommended is greatly increased.

More recently, two studies were reported that have shown that statin use reduces the risk of dementia and could be recommended for the prevention of Alzheimer's disease.[14] The experts are beginning to think that statins may be in order for most people over the age of 50. My conclusion: statins are our friends.

Statins Are the New Aspirin

During the November 2001 American Heart Association conference in Anaheim, California, a study of a statin drug and its power to reduce cholesterol and prevent heart attacks and strokes was revealed.[15] Researchers call the findings definitive, because of the size and length of the study; 20,000 patients in England and Scotland, men and women ages 40 to 80, were followed for an average of five years. All the subjects were at risk for cardiovascular disease. Significantly, the findings of this study indicated that statin drug therapy can reduce heart attacks and strokes by as

---

[13] NIH, National Cholesterol Educational Program. Report May 2001. www.nhlbi.nih.gov/guidelines/cholesterol.
[14] "Beyond Cholesterol: New Uses for Statins," *American Medical News,* June 18, 2001, www.amednews.com.
[15] American Heart Association Scientific Sessions 2001, Anaheim CA, www.americanheart.org.

much as one third, not only in people with high cholesterol, but in persons with other risk factors, such as diabetes.

The findings have strong implications for public health and would indicate the use of statins for twice the number of persons currently taking them. The specific statin drug involved in the study was *simvastatin* (marketed by Merck as Zocor); however, researchers state that the findings would likely apply to all the drugs in this category.

After a decade of research and clinical experience, we're pretty sure that statin drugs (Lipitor, Zocor, Mevacor, etc.) are effective therapies for managing lipid levels in persons at risk for heart ailments. But are they cost-effective? Lipitor, for example, can cost a patient over $100 a month. Is it worth it? Researchers have a way of measuring cost-effectiveness, and in two recent studies they report that the statins are indeed cost-effective for secondary prevention for patients with known heart disease, but not so as primary prevention among patients not known to have heart disease.[16] They calculate the cost against a unit of value which they call a "QALY" —standing for quality-adjusted life-year. Statins cost $45,000 per QALY for secondary prevention and are considered cost-effective. In the epidemiological surveys used as the basis of these findings, ratios of $50,000 per QALY and greater were found among primary prevention groups of subjects and are not considered cost-effective.

The researchers then compared ratios in other preventive therapies. Here are some examples:

- An annual mammogram for a woman age 55-65 is rated at $150,000 per QALY. (Not cost-effective)
- An angioplasty in patients with only mild angina is rated at $112,000 per QALY. (Not cost-effective)
- Single vessel angioplasty in patients with severe angina rated at $10,000 per QALY. (Cost effective)

As this measuring calculation indicates, the more the therapy benefits the patient, the more it is valued, and the more it is cost-effective. Were there any lingering questions about the appropriateness of prescribing a regimen of lipid lowering drugs for heart disease patients, these findings appear to resolve them.

---

[16] Prosser, Lisa, A., et al., "Cost Effectiveness Of Cholesterol-lowering Therapies According To Selected Patient Characteristics," *Annals of Internal Medicine*, May 16, 2000.

HOPE: From Trials to Clinical Benefits

Reports continue to be published in the medical journals of new findings and analyses of data from the HOPE Trials. I've referred to HOPE many times in discussions on guidelines for ACE inhibitor therapy. HOPE stands for *Heart Outcomes Prevention Evaluation*. It is a project conducted by the Department of Cardiology of McMaster University (Hamilton, Ontario, Canada) that began in 1996.

There was an important HOPE development in June 2000 when the Cardiovascular and Renal Drugs Advisory Committee[17] of the FDA recommended the ACE inhibitor *ramipril* (generic name) for prevention of heart attack and stroke in high-risk patients. Indeed, since results of HOPE were first presented at a meeting of the European Society of Cardiology in Barcelona in August in 1999,[18] researchers and clinicians have had their attention focused on this landmark study.

Described as a "simple, randomized trial," it aims at learning whether an angiotensin-converting enzyme (ACE) inhibitor, in this case, ramipril, combined with the natural antioxidant vitamin E, would be effective in preventing heart attacks and strokes. Ten milligrams of the drug and appropriate dosages of the vitamin (and placebos) were administered orally once a day to over 9,000 patients through hospitals and doctors offices in North and South America and Europe. The subjects were men and women 55 years old and older who had heart disease and were at risk for cardiovascular events. Among these, 36 percent were diabetics. Although the trial was scheduled for the duration of five years, it was interrupted after four and one-half years because there was clear evidence of risk reduction in the ramipril group, and the researchers could not ethically deny those benefits to patients in the placebo group.

According to the reports, there were positive results evident in the first year of the trial, and those effects continued in the follow up years. Compared to the control (placebo) group, the drug was found to lower the risk of heart attack by 22 percent and the risk of stroke by 33 percent. No positive effect of vitamin E has been observed, yet this section of the trials is continuing. All the subjects in the trial experienced the benefits of the

[17] Federal Drug Administration. Search: "Ramipril" at
www.fda.gov/cder/audiences/acspage/Cardiovascularcharter1.html.
[18] Yusuf, S., Sleight, P., " The HOPE Study (Heart Outcomes Prevention Evaluation," *European Society of Cardiology*, XXI Annual Congress in Barcelona 1999, www.escardio.org.

ramipril, which analysts believe to be a slowing down of progress of athrosclerosis as well as a neutralizing of plaques already formed in the coronary and cerebral arteries. In other words, the drug halts the advance of heart disease. In addition, while the drug did not impede the development of kidney disease in diabetics, it seems to have prevented the onset of diabetes in the trial population.

For many years, ACE inhibitor drugs like ramipril have been administered to patients to control blood pressure. The findings of the HOPE trials show that ramipril has even greater benefits in protecting against deleterious effects of cardiovascular diseases and against renal failure in diabetics. In the words of an editorial in the *New England Journal of Medicine*,[19] "the results of the HOPE study make it clear that the benefits of ACE inhibitors—in this case, ramipril—exceed our expectations. It is overly simplistic to label these drugs vasodilators. They appear to have effects on the vasculature, heart, and kidneys that go far beyond their rather small blood-pressure-lowering effects." HOPE is a major advance in clinical care of heart disease victims. The anticoagulant benefits of aspirin plus cholesterol-lowering drugs and the ACE inhibitor ramipril (marketed under the brand name Altace) present a potent offense in the battle against America's number one killer.

Good Ol' Reliable Aspirin

Just about everyone at risk for cardiovascular disease should take low dose aspirin daily, yet doctors estimate that only one out of every three people who would benefit from aspirin actually take it. Numerous investigations have shown the almost magical property of this inexpensive drug in preventing cardiovascular problems. In a study reported in the *Archives of Internal Medicine*,[20] Harvard researchers analyzed data from the classic Physician Health Study, and found that volunteers who conscientiously adhered to an aspirin regimen for five years had 51 percent reduction in their risk of heart attack, compared with their counterparts who

[19] Rosenthal, N., "High Hopes for the Heart," (Editorial), *New England Journal of Medicine,* June 7, 2001.
[20] Cook, Nancy R., et al., "Self-Selected Post-trial Aspirin Use and Subsequent Cardiovascular Disease and Mortality in the Physicians' Health Study," *Archives of Internal Medicine,* April 10, 2000.

took a placebo.[21] Those participants who reported poor adherence to the aspirin regimen had a nonsignificant reduction in their risk of heart attack.

This is just one of dozens of studies on the benefits of aspirin. Besides preventing heart attacks and angina, aspirin taken within 24 hours of the onset of heart attack will increase the chance of survival by 23 percent. For those patients who have had a heart attack, it reduces the risk by 50 percent. It also significantly reduces the risk of stroke. Aspirin works by blocking the production of prostagladins, which causes the clumping of blood cells called platelets resulting in the formation of blood clots. These clots block the flow of blood to the heart and cause heart attack; or, should they form in the neck or head, will trigger a stroke. Studies also indicate that aspirin may be a powerful weapon in fighting other diseases, such as cancer of the colon, esophagus, stomach, and rectum. It even improves brain function in people with dementias.

Who should take aspirin? Men over 40 and women over 50 who have one or more of the major risk factors for heart disease, such as high cholesterol, obesity, a family history of early heart attack, or who smoke. In a review of 300 studies from all over the world, researchers reported that aspirin benefits anyone suffering from any vascular disease; that is, any disease where the underlying mechanism involves closing of the circulatory system with a clot. The findings held true regardless of age, race, or history of diabetes or hypertension. Keep in mind I recommend these rules for taking aspirin:

- Take one half an adult aspirin or a baby aspirin daily. More is not better. At higher doses, aspirin may be less effective in combating heart disease.
- Be sure you are taking aspirin, not one of the other painkillers such as acetaminophen (Tylenol) or ibuprofen.
- If aspirin upsets your stomach, take the coated type.
- Most people can take low dose aspirin without any adverse affects. However, do not take aspirin if:
  - You are allergic to it.
  - You have high blood pressure, kidney or liver disease, or a family history of cerebral aneurysm.

---

[21] Physicians Health Study (ongoing since 1982), of data collected from over 20,000 physician-subjects. Directed by renowned epidemiologist Dr. Charles Hennekens, Professor of Medicine at Harvard Medical School. This study established, among other things, the health benefits of daily aspirin therapy.

- You are taking an anticoagulant.
- You have an iron or folic acid deficiency or a vitamin B-12 malabsorption problem.

Experts suggest that potential heart attack victims always keep a supply of aspirin nearby, including on planes, in backpacks, or in cars when traveling. They also urge that aspirin not be substituted for the proper management of other heart disease risk factors. In other words, even though you are on a low dose aspirin regimen, you must still eat a low fat diet, exercise, lose weight, and stop smoking.

MDs Prescribe Too Few Drugs

According to reports presented at the November 1999 meeting of the American Heart Association,[22] physicians are not prescribing an adequate amount of drugs to their heart patients. ACE inhibitors, beta-blockers, and warfarin are all drugs that should be more widely used and that can reduce the number of deaths from heart disease.

ACE Inhibitors
In addition to their effectiveness in combating hypertension, ACE inhibitors are beneficial to patients with congestive heart failure, which currently affects 4.7 million Americans. These drugs help a weakened heart pump blood. Yet, according to the new investigation, doctors prescribed ACE inhibitors to only approximately 25 percent of patients who could probably benefit from them.

In analyzing a representative sample of 1,529 doctor's visits by patients with congestive heart failure, investigators discovered that, as might be expected, cardiologists were the most likely to prescribe ACE inhibitors. In fact, they gave them to their patients twice as often as other physicians. Doctors in urban areas were more likely to prescribe them than doctors in rural or suburban areas. The drugs were more likely to be prescribed to privately insured patients (39%) versus those with no private insurance (24%). The use of ACE inhibitors did not increase between 1989 and 1994, which researchers believe means that many physicians have not yet gotten the message about the benefits of these drugs. They

---

[22] American Heart Association Scientific Sessions November 1999. Search: "High doses of ACE inhibitors . . ." at AHA website www.americanheart.org.

38

also believe that it indicates physicians are not paying enough attention to strategies to prevent heart disease.

Beta-Blockers

Beta-blockers are very effective at reducing angina, hypertension, and the risk of a second heart attack. Indeed, they have been found to reduce mortality by 25 percent after a heart attack. A second new study reveals that in a group of California heart attack patients, only 37.7 percent were prescribed beta-blocker therapy at the time of discharge from the hospital.

Beta-blockers do have significant side effects, yet the researchers claim that if the drugs are prescribed to all heart attack victims who can tolerate them, a large number of lives would be saved. Beta-blockers are particularly useful for heart attack patients who do not have an angioplasty or bypass surgery to unblock their clogged coronary arteries. If these patients take beta-blockers, they are three times less likely to die than those who do not.

Some of the side effects of beta-blockers are depression, sexual dysfunction, and tiredness. The investigators suggested that one of the reasons physicians may not be prescribing this drug is that they overestimate the side effects. More research is needed, they say, to determine why beta-blockers are so underutilized and how to get physicians to use them more aggressively.

Warfarin

Warfarin reduces the risk of a recurrent stroke. In reviewing the charts of 635 patients admitted to a hospital in Connecticut, investigators found only 50 percent of patients in the hospital with a stroke were prescribed the drug.

Drugs have a lifesaving role in combating heart disease, particularly in more serious cases. As new therapies develop, all doctors must keep up with the research.

Improved Drug Therapy Aids Management of Diabetes

If unchecked, diabetes can quadruple a person's risk of heart disease and stroke, cause blindness, amputation, kidney disease, and nerve damage. These dire consequences of diabetes are not inevitable, however. The good news is that if patients take control of their disease, they can prevent and even reverse these deadly complications. The goal of all therapy for diabetes is to maintain blood sugar levels as close to normal as possible. A breakthrough study released in 1993, called the *Diabetes Control and Complications Trial*, revealed that diabetic patients who maintain tight control over their blood sugar levels (called glycemic control) reduce the risk of diabetic eye disease by 76 percent, the risk of nerve damage by 60 percent, the risk of diabetic kidney disease by 50 percent, and the risk of cardiovascular disease by 35 percent.[23]

As a result of these findings, doctors and diabetes educators have been working with patients to help them implement the many techniques available to keep blood sugar levels under control. For patients, this requires organization, effort, and discipline. Unfortunately, too many do not face up to this early on in the course of their disease, and by the time they come to my office the diabetes has wreaked its damage on their body.

Diabetics must begin their fight against the disease by monitoring their blood glucose at home. The cornerstone of diabetes management and glycemic control consists of diet, weight loss, and exercise. If patients ignore these behavioral requirements for controlling diabetes, the other treatments probably will not be very effective. Most Type 2 diabetics—the majority of people with the disease—can achieve glycemic control with oral medications rather than insulin injections, if they are conscientious about the lifestyle requirements. Type 1 diabetics, however, will require insulin injections; but with behavioral changes, oral medication, and careful monitoring, they should be able to decrease the amount and number of injections.

Oral Medications

In the last decade, several oral medications have been discovered that can be used successfully in the treatment of diabetes. These drugs aid in the management of the diabetes; they do not cure it. Up until 1994, only one type of oral medication was available for diabetes, *sulfonylurea drugs*. These reduce blood glucose levels by stimulating the pancreas to increase insulin production. This helps get more glucose out of the blood and into the cells. Doctors generally prescribe the sulfonylurea drugs for those who have had Type 2 diabetes for less than five years and do not use insulin. The problem with this medication, however, is that some people don't respond to it at all, and others may respond for a few years and then stop.

---

[23] Diabetes Control and Complications Trial (DCCT) is a clinical study conducted from 1983 to 1993 by the National Institute of Diabetes and Digestive and Kidney Diseases (NIDDK), www.niddk.nih.gov/health/diabetes/pubs/dcctl/dcct.htm.

Sulfonylurea drugs do not work with diabetics who have few functioning beta cells, the pancreatic cells that produce insulin.

Glucophage (metformin), approved for the U.S. market in 1994, offered a giant leap forward in treating diabetes. It usually reduces the level of blood glucose by 25 to 30 percent and is successful in about 80 percent of people who take it. Glucophage works by suppressing the liver's release of stored glucose. An added benefit of the drug is that it helps with weight loss. Not everyone can take Glucophage, however, because it causes lactic acidosis in people with chronic respiratory disease, heart, kidney or liver disease, or alcoholism.

Precose (acarbose), available since 1996, is taken with the first bite of the meal, and it blocks the action of certain enzymes that help digest carbohydrates. By blocking their digestion, less glucose gets into the blood. It is therefore useful in controlling the spikes in glucose levels that occur after a meal.

Rezulin (troglitazone) came on the market for Type 2 diabetics in 1996. It helps the body use its own insulin more efficiently and enables those using injectable insulin to cut their dosage by half on average. In about 15 percent of cases, patients may eliminate insulin altogether. The initial enthusiasm for Rezulin has been tempered by reports of liver problems in patients taking it. I believe this can be an excellent drug, but the physician must monitor its usage very carefully. Because of its risks, it is recommended only for diabetics whose glucose levels remain poorly controlled despite proper diet, exercise, and the use of other medications.

Prandin is the newest drug for diabetics. Given before meals, it quickly raises the insulin level at the time it is needed. These drugs may be used alone, but doctors have begun to prescribe them in combination, because they attack the problems of controlling glucose levels in different ways.

None of these drugs are a panacea. All cause side effects, ranging from mild to severe. For those who do need insulin, they must determine how much they need and how often, working with their doctor or a diabetes educator as well as through trial and error. The idea is to imitate the normal flow of insulin from the pancreas. Achieving this is different for everyone, depending on the diet, weight, activity level, stress level, and the body's individual response. Those using insulin must be alert to the hazards and warning signs of low blood sugar, which, if ignored, can result in coma or death. Alternatives to injections include implantable insulin pumps and, soon to be available, inhalable insulin.

Patients Are Not Taking Their Medicine

Patients' noncompliance with treatment recommended by their doctor has become a serious medical problem. As more and better drugs and other therapies become available, medical professionals are dismayed to discover that those patients who could greatly benefit from treatment are just not going along with the program. Among heart patients, not only are many of them not making the lifestyle changes that have been proven to help their heart disease, in many cases they are not even taking medicines that have proven effective and are known to many save lives.

Bad habits after bypass

For example, the majority of women who have heart bypass surgery do not change the unhealthy habits that contributed to their condition in the first place. According to studies, six months after the surgery, 59 percent of the women who had undergone bypass operations did not have their high blood pressure under control; 85 percent had higher than recommended cholesterol levels. Both of these conditions can be readily changed by diet, exercise, and medication. If they are not altered, the risk of further disease is greatly magnified. Ten percent of women undergoing bypass surgery even continued to smoke afterwards!

Diabetics & Aspirin

As another example, people with diabetes are at high risk for heart attack and stroke. Research shows that an aspirin a day is very effective in preventing these deadly events; yet, only one in five diabetics take aspirin daily. Even among those diabetics who actually have heart disease, only 37 percent reported using aspirin regularly.

MDs not doing their job?

Medical professionals are "doing a terrible job" in educating patients to the importance of following their treatment regimen, said Dr. Richard Paternak, director of cardiology at Massachusetts General Hospital, during a recent American Heart Association meeting.

He gave as an example the failure of many heart patients to continue taking the very effective statin drugs to reduce cholesterol. We know that these medications may slash the risk of heart attack and stroke by more than 50 percent. Yet only about half of the patients prescribed these drugs have continued to take them a year later. After two years, only 15 percent of patients are still taking them. Other studies have found a similar pattern with blood pressure medication.

No Confidence in Drugs?

It almost seems as if these patients have a death wish. Why won't they take their medicine? For some, it is that they don't have confidence that the drugs will work. Perhaps their doctors have not explained why they should take the drugs or how patients have fared in clinical trials. When individuals have a procedure such as bypass surgery, they often assume that it has fixed their problem and they don't have to worry anymore. Again, doctors may fail to communicate to them that they are still very much at risk. The U.S. health care system focuses too strongly on crisis care, says Dr. Paternak, attending to patients when they require hospital care, then losing track of them once they leave the hospital. Patients need continuing medical advice, education, and followup from their doctors.

Chapter Three
Invasive Solutions

Angioplasty Is Here to Stay

Every once in a while, the question arises among health care practitioners as to whether *percutaneous coronary intervention* (PCI) or angioplasty is really worth the trouble. After all, upwards of 20 percent of the procedures have to be repeated because their effect is not lasting. Today there are powerful drugs, which can have a similar positive effect on arteries.

PCI, or angioplasty, is a procedure in which the physician inserts a catheter (intervenes) through a puncture under the skin (percutaneous) to clear blockages in the arteries of the heart (coronary). The buildup of fatty and sticky substances or plaque causes these blockages. Different techniques and instruments may be used to remove plaque. Sometimes a tiny balloon is inflated at the end of the catheter to push the plaque aside; sometimes a blade or a laser beam is used to break up the plaque. In some of these procedures a stent or plastic tubing is inserted to hold the artery open for the flow of blood.

In a Commentary in the *Journal of Invasive Cardiology*,[24] Dr. William S. Weintraub of Emory University assumes that PCI is here to stay and, indeed, "physicians' sworn moral obligation to serve their patients' interests mandates a social contact to use this service wisely and with optimum patient outcome." Dr. Weintraub's analysis notes that PCI is a good treatment for angina and is lifesaving in the setting of acute myocardial infarction; that is, it is appropriate for preventing a second heart attack, although not as preventive therapy for patients without symptoms. In his review of research on this procedure over the twenty years of its use, he reports that it is more successful when performed in large institutions rather than in small. He cites the recommendation of the American College of Cardiology that institutions should perform a minimum of 200

---

[24] Weintraub, Wiliam, "Commentary," *Journal of Invasive Cardiology*, November, 2000.

procedures per year. In the context of moral obligating and social contract, which Dr. Weintraub establishes, it could be argued that restricting angioplasties to fewer institutions would deprive some patients of its benefits. The question remains open, but in the meantime continuing education programs by the American College of Cardiology and the American Heart Association aim at helping smaller institutions improve their performance.

In the United States today, there are over 500,000 PCI procedures performed yearly, at a cost in excess of $5 billion. For some victims of heart disease, this service is replacing cardiac surgery as the most commonly used technique for repairing coronary arteries. To aid in fulfilling the social contract Dr. Weintraub recognizes, there are currently 300 catheterization laboratories that perform PCIs participating in a study conducted by the American College of Cardiology. The study is expected to produce data that will facilitate the evaluation of the quality of PCI services and improve PCI so that it may be available to everyone who needs it.

Angioplasty in Community Hospitals

When a blockage in one of your coronary arteries requires that you undergo angioplasty, you are asked to sign a consent form permitting the hospital's surgical team to perform a bypass graph operation should it be indicated in the course of the angioplasty. State Health Department regulations require that during the angioplasty there be a bypass surgical team standing by. New York regulations also require special qualifications for a hospital to perform angioplasties; these are Heart Centers. But all this could change. Some scientists looking at the high number of heart attacks occurring in the U.S. each year (1.2 million), conducted a trial in which they compared the outcomes of angioplasties performed in community hospital emergency rooms on heart attack victims with application of clot-busting drugs, the accepted therapy in these life and death situations. The drugs are a class called tissue plasminogen activators or TPAs, and they have been highly successful in treating heart attack victims in emergencies. Could on the spot angioplasties do better? The statistical data says yes.

The research was lead by Dr. Thomas Aversano of John's Hopkins and reported in the *Journal of the American Medical Association*[25] in an article titled "Thrombolytic Therapy vs. Primary Percutaneous Coronary

---

[25] Aversano, T., et al., "Percutaneous Coronary Intervention for Myocardial Infarction in Patients Presenting to Hospitals Without On-site Cardiac Surgery," *Journal of the American Medical Association (JAMA)*, April 17, 2002.

Intervention for Myocardial Infarction in Patients Presenting to Hospitals Without On-site Cardiac Surgery." Dr. Aversano's research was conducted in noncardiac center hospitals mainly around Boston and Baltimore and named the Atlantic C-PORT study, standing for Cardiovascular Patient Outcomes Research Team. It involved 451 heart attack patients over a three-year period from 1996 to 1999. Half were randomly assigned angioplasty treatment; the others received drugs. In a six-month intervening period, the angioplasty patients fared better, not by dramatic numbers, but consistently. These findings confirmed what earlier studies had concluded: heart attack victims do better when given emergency angioplasty than when treated with drugs, and this can be done in community hospital settings. Our strategy for treating heart attack victims could be upgraded if community hospitals were prepared to perform emergency angioplasties.

In the Cath Lab with Vice President Cheney

Those one in four American who are affected by heart disease paid special attention to the charts and diagrams in the news reports of Vice President Dick Cheney's hospitalization in February 2001. Reporters did an excellent job describing the effects of atherosclerosis (heart disease) and in explaining therapies used to address it in the "cath-lab." The cath-lab is the surgical unit where a catheter, a long narrow (1 cm in diameter) tubing, is used to access a coronary artery in angioplasty procedures. Those colorful illustrations in the media of the Vice President's occluded artery and of the stent used to open it up were magnificent teaching aids. Hopefully, all Americans who followed this story renewed their resolve to take appropriate measures to prevent the deleterious effects of cardiovascular disease in their own lives.

The Vice President, having previously had an angioplasty to open a blocked artery in his heart, said he was experiencing episodes of unstable angina (angina pain which occurs without any physical exertion and doesn't go away during rest). This happens because the heart doesn't get the oxygen it needs when the blood flow in the coronary artery is partially closed off. This is called *restenosis*—meaning the occlusion has come back again after an artery has been cleared by angioplasty. The angioplasty performed on the Vice President the year before included the insertion of a stent, which is a mesh tubing made of metal (in some cases, plastic). The stent is intended to keep the artery open once the blockage is cleared. Today over 80 percent of angioplasties involve the insertion of a stent.

47

Stents: The State of the Art

Following the Vice President's medical emergency and the controversy about the use of stenting in angioplasties that it set off, there has been a rash of articles in the medical journals discussing various aspects of stents. The question arose as to whether it should have been treated with radiation to improve its effectiveness—the brachytherapy procedure. Listed below are some of the discussions of stenting that followed in the literature:

- Should the placement of a stent (flexible metal or plastic tubing that holds open an occluded artery) be favored over bypassing the occlusion with a surgical procedure? Which solution is best? Studies conducted in Europe and in the United States recently have shown advantages for both approaches. The stent procedure is less costly, except that it often needs to be repeated, bringing its overall cost close to that of bypass surgery. A comparison of mortality rates is inconclusive. In the opinion of one researcher, physicians would be best advised to make an assessment in each individual case, particularly when many coronary arteries are involved. It might even be appropriate to combine the two procedures.
- The Cordis Corporation, a division of Johnson & Johnson, is a prominent manufacturer of stents. It offers designs using a variety of materials, different diameters, and different lengths; and the company is developing new and specialized products all the time. Their latest is a stent (*Bx Velocity*™) made for "treatment of abrupt or threatened closure of coronary arteries." Typically, this stent was tested in more than 150 patients in medical centers around the country. It is said to feature enhanced flexibility for getting around tight turns and minimal surface friction during insertion.
- In a narrowly defined study examining the outcome data of 16,000 angioplasty procedures during a two-year period in the 1990s, research analysts found that when stents were used in the procedures the in-hospital survival rate was better than when stents were not used. Stents were associated with a significant reduction of in-hospital mortality, compared with balloon procedures. The risk of emergency coronary bypass also was reduced by stenting. This report,[26] out of the

---

[26] Kimmel, Stephen E., et al. "Effects of Coronary Stents on Cardiovascular Outcomes in Broad-Based Clinical Practice," *Archives of Internal Medicine,* September 25, 2000.

University of Pennsylvania School of Medicine, offers strong support for the uses of stents, common now in about 80 percent of all angioplasties.

Stents and Radiation

Reporters solicited commentary on the Vice President's situation story from cardiologists in the major hospitals in Washington, Boston, and New York. Some of them felt V.P. Cheney should have had a radiation treatment called brachytherapy at the time they inserted the stent. In this therapy, tiny radioactive seeds or pellets are deployed through the catheter directly to the treatment site. The radiation kills certain cells and prevents scar tissue from growing. With the use of *beta* radiation, physicians can remain at the patient's side during the treatment. The radiation seeds do not remain in the body and the total body exposure is no greater than that received during a chest Xray. Trials have shown that irradiated stents are much less likely to occlude again. Radiation treated stents reduce the risk of restenosis as much as 66 percent, say researchers.

But brachytherapy is a new therapy and not available in all hospitals. It was not available at George Washington University Hospital, where V.P. Cheney was treated. Physicians there, however, hold the opinion along with others that brachytherapy is only called for after a stent has failed more than once. If, as most cardiac experts believe, there is a 40 percent chance of the Vice President's artery clogging up again, the next step might be the radiation pellets.

Other Options

Cordis Corporation coats stents with a medication to make them more artery-friendly. This has had good results in small trials, and it is said to have some advantages over irradiated stents. A Japanese medical center has conducted trials with a stent made of biodegradable material. The rationale for this stent, which could be completely absorbed by the body in 18 months, is that it eliminates the risk of clots that metal stents might trigger over the long term. Another stent coated with a solvent-like substance had positive results in German pilot studies.

Despite the number of studies done with these innovations so far, it is not clear, say researchers, that coated stents will be the long-term solution to restenosis problems. What molecular biologists are looking to next is *myogenisis*— the replacement of scarred myocardium (artery walls) through injections of cultured peripheral muscle cells—growing new coronary arteries. More about this biogenetic approach follows in this section.

The experts know that damage is done to coronary arteries not only by an infarction (heart attack), but also to a limited extent by the surgeries and therapies we employ to correct it. Angioplasties and stents are intrusive and inflict trauma on the arterial walls, leaving scar tissue in their wake. All the more reason why the best approach to cardiovascular disease is an aggressive program of prevention.

The Technology for Treating Tachycardia: A heart that beats too fast.

Our Vice President, Dick Cheney, has referred to himself as a "symbol of American cardiac technology." Indeed, since his health problems came to national attention, health educators have had many opportunities to explain some common procedures for ailing hearts.

In this discussion we will encounter two cardiac problems, *ventricular tachycardia* and *ventricular fibrillation* and devices used in their diagnosis and treatment. Heart disease, we have learned, is chronic. If your constitution is disposed to it, it can begin early—as early as your teen years. That's why it is so important to see that children do not get into bad diet habits, especially if there is some presence of heart disease in the family. The disease may persist for decades and, with each coronary event (heart attack) one survives, the heart is damaged irreparably. Little by little its function becomes weaker and weaker. The nature of heart disease is a narrowing of the arteries in the heart and arteries of the body. This is caused by the buildup of plaques, gummy substances, fats and the like, that stick to the arteries' walls. The medical name for this condition is *atherosclerosis*.

On more than one occasion, the Vice President had to have one of his coronary arteries cleared out by an angioplasty procedure and a plastic mess stent inserted to keep it open. The last time the problem was different. His doctors, ever watchful of his health, asked him to wear a *Holter monitor* for 24 hours in order to learn if there were any irregularities or deficiencies in his heart function. The Holter monitor is commonly prescribed for patients who have suffered heart damage. It is a virtual portable electrocardiograph machine that records heart rhythms. In setting it up, electrodes are placed on the patient's chest and connected to a recording box strapped around the patient's waist that can be hidden under

50

clothing. Heart rate is monitored and recorded on tape throughout the day's activities and during sleep. The patient is advised to keep a diary (V.P. Cheney did this.) so that daily physical activities can be compared to the data recorded on the tape. A Holter monitor is usually put on in the hospital; it takes only 10 or 15 minutes to set it up and no special preparation is required of the patient. It is painless, of course, and only moderately inconvenient or uncomfortable, say, at night in bed, plus you are unable to take a shower.

When they read the data on the Vice President's Holter tape, his doctors saw evidence of several instances of *ventricular tachycardia*. The entry in the medical dictionary is so clear and precise in explaining ventricular tachycardia that I quote it here at length:

> Ventricular tachycardia is an arrhythmia [irregular rhythm] that originates in the pumping heart's chambers, or the ventricles. It is usually seen in patients who have damaged ventricular chambers, frequently in the aftermath of a heart attack. Scar tissue in the ventricles will alter many local electrical properties and set up conditions favorable to formation of a local electrical circuit. Under specific circumstances, the circuit can be activated leading to a rapid arrhythmia arising from a single spot within the pumping chambers. [27]

Although they may last only an instant and are not felt, a heart with signs of ventricular tachycardias requires treatment. There is the danger that they may lead to *ventricular fibrillation*. This is immediately life threatening, because the pumping mechanism is so out of whack that the heart begins to quiver, disrupting the flow of blood to the rest of the body. Electric shock that interrupts the irregular rhythms of the heart and resets its normal rhythm is the emergency treatment for ventricular fibrillation. The device used is a defibrillator; it stops the quivering, stops the fibrillations. Ventricular tachycardia, when it does not lead to an emergency condition, may be treated with medications.

In V.P. Cheney's case, his doctors elected to insert an *implantable cardioverter defibrillator* (ICD) in his chest just below his left collarbone. Implantable means that a small incision is made and the pager-size electric device is placed under the skin. The ICD consists of a pulse generator with a sealed lithium battery and an electronic circuitry package. A tiny wire or

---

[27] The Arrhythmia Service, St Luke's-Roosevelt Hospital, New York NY, www.arrhythmia.org.

lead from the ICD is inserted into the aorta (the large vessel delivering blood out of the heart to other parts of the body) and then threaded down into the problem ventricle. The pulse generator produces the electrical signals that affect the heart's rhythm. Today's ultra-sophisticated ICD functions as both a pacemaker and a defibrillator. It has the capability to receive and respond to signals that are sent by the heart and can be preprogrammed for a certain healthy heart rate range. When the patient's heart rate goes below or above that range, the ICD kicks in to correct it. The surgery is done with a local anesthesia in about an hour's time, and the patient can usually go home the same day.

ICDs have been in use since 1980. More than 150,000 Americans are currently beneficiaries of this technology, which has been described as having "an ER in the chest." It literally prevents sudden death by a heart attack and is usually prescribed for heart disease patients who have suffered heart attacks and therefore are at very serious risk. When its defibrillation function kicks in, the patient may feel an explosive jolt in the chest. But, say the scientist-caregivers, that's a small price to pay for the ICD's lifesaving effect.

Report Is Positive on Heart Surgery for the Elderly

Most research done on heart disease does not include in its sample enough patients over the age of 75 to give any clear indication as to the value of specific therapies for the elderly. Often the elderly are suffering one or more ailments in addition to heart disease, which complicates the question of whether to offer them heart surgery to relieve their symptoms. At The 23rd Congress of the European Society of Cardiology the question was addressed and given a positive answer. It featured presentations on research projects conducted by scientists from every European country as well as the United States, Canada, Australia, and New Zealand. In one of these projects, the TIME trial (Trial of Invasive vs. Medical therapy in the Elderly) data was presented showing that the elderly, persons over 75, could benefit by invasive therapies—angioplasty or bypass surgery— if they were not responding to medications for their disease.

A group of 301 patients, average age 80, were followed over a period of five years in the Swiss study, approximately one-half receiving medical treatments, and one-half receiving appropriate invasive procedures. Those in the latter section of the study experienced a very significantly lower incidence of cardiac events as well as relief of symptoms such as angina and lack of stamina. While there is risk involved in offering invasive procedures to these elderly patients, the study indicates that the risk-benefit ratio is in their favor. That is, while invasive therapies may not effect longevity, they can greatly improve quality of life. It was noted by one commentator at this presentation, that since the study was initiated more than five years ago the patients in the medical section would not have had the benefit of the most recent and powerful drugs developed to treat heart disease—such as the ace inhibitor ramipril (Altace), and the statins (Lipitor, Zocor, etc.).

Better Heart Surgery

The American Heart Association sponsors 15 or more professional conferences on cardiovascular disease and related subjects every year. Some of the conferences focus exclusively on specific aspects of disease, such as hypertension, prevention, and obesity. In November 2001, at AHA's 2001 Scientific Sessions in Anaheim California, more than 300 presentations were made by researchers from around the globe, and over 4000 abstracts of studies were submitted.[28] These findings covered the latest research in a myriad of areas that included stem cell therapies, acupuncture, heart disease in children (Kawasaki disease), as well as drugs for treatments approved or awaiting FDA approval.

A review of published materials of the conference proceedings turned up subjects already familiar to followers of cardiovascular disease news (e.g., a study on the apparent benefits of moderate alcohol consumption for heart disease sufferers). There are also studies on experimental therapies whose application in clinical practice may be far off in the future. Nonetheless, all the research is fresh, all advance our understanding of cardiovascular disease and provides useful information for managing our heart health, which we have come to know is "in our own hands."

Three reports presented ways of improving heart surgery and its outcomes. Surgeon-scientists tested and found safe, better methods for suturing the replacement veins in bypass surgery. In one technique, a stainless steel clip device is used to secure the blood vessels at either end of the bypass. The other technique uses adhesives to bond the grafted blood vessels. So far this latter method has only been used in animals,

---

[28] American Heart Association Scientific Sessions 2001, Anaheim CA, www.medscape.com/viewprogram/180.

where the adhesives were found to fully seal the blood vessels and allow excellent blood flow.

The major advantage of both techniques is in reducing, by more than half (5 to 2 minutes) the time it takes for the surgeon to hand stitch the grafts, while the heart is stopped and blood circulation is dependent on the heart-lung machine. The scientists see a time when these techniques may eliminate the heart-lung machine altogether, achieving an operation with less chance of harmful aftereffects. Patients taking the vitamin supplement coenzyme Q10 before coronary bypass surgery were reported in one abstract to have shorter postoperative stays, because of less heart muscle damage and better heart function. Coenzyme Q10 enhances cell energy. It is often given to heart failure patients.

Heart Briefs

To Angiogram or Not to Angiogram

Physicians order thousands of angiograms each year for patients who complain of chest pain. The angiogram consists of injecting a transparent dye into the heart by way of a catheter inserted into an artery in the groin; it is passed upward to the heart and then viewed in real time on a video screen and later on film. The angiogram is an excellent and decisive method for determining a heart's condition.

The question arises, however, as to what steps to take if the heart appears healthy. Was the angiogram, which involves a certain level of risk, appropriate and useful after all? A doctor writing in *Medscape Cardiology* argues that it is indeed safe and that the arteriographers who perform the angiogram ought to consult with the patient's physician as a means of continuing the pursuit of a definitive diagnosis.[29] While the patient's symptom has been determined to be *noncardiac chest pain,* there are many other causes of chest pain that should be explored. "The assumption that noncardiac chest pain is not serious," writes Dr. J. William Hurst, "is not correct." Angiographers ought to be sufficiently concerned about solving a patient's problem that they share their views about the cause of the pain with the referring physician, since as he points out, their role is more than that of a technician.

---

[29] Hurst, J. Willis, "Further Thoughts on Diagnosing Noncardiac Chest Pain," *Medscape Cardiology,* www.medscape.com/viewarticle/403290.

Operating on a Beating Heart

There have been reports in the press lately of heart bypass patients suffering memory loss years after their surgery. In a study referred to in the online medical news source *WebMD*, patients were said to suffer decline in short-term memory, attention span, concentration, and language comprehension.[30] Experts believe that the heart-lung machine employed to take over the heart's pumping function during bypass surgery is the cause of these aftereffects. For this reason, many surgeons are turning to off-pump techniques, which allows them to operate on the beating heart without the heart-lung machine. The irony is that is was the heart-lung machine, invented in the early 1970s, that made human heart surgery possible and successful. The new off-pump method involves the use of mechanical stabilizers attached to the heart around the area to be bypassed, that keeps that area still during the surgery. Only about 20 percent of bypass surgeries are performed off-pump, although patients are now being offered their choice of either of these methods. In addition to avoiding the aforementioned aftereffects, off-pump bypass surgery is said to reduce the amount of blood loss and shorten the hospital stay. Statistics also show a slightly better survival rate when the off-pump technique is used.

Repaired Hearts, New Hearts

Two major advances in what we know about the human heart were announced in 2001. In California, surgeons injected muscle cells from the patient's bicep into the back of his heart where it had been damaged by two heart attacks. When a heart attack occurs, the *infracted*, or overstuffed blood vessels in the heart burst destroying cell function in that area. Cells functioning properly will multiply and restore the damage. In the California procedure, it took only three minutes to inject the bicep muscle cells during a bypass operation. It will take time to find out whether the bicep cells function properly and rebuild the damaged area of the patient's heart.

The second advance, reported almost concurrently with the California news, was the announcement from a researcher at New York Medical College in Valhalla NY, that he had succeeded in regrowing heart cells. It has always been believed that the cells of the heart muscle do not have the regenerative capacity of cells in other organs of the body. Dr. Piero Anversa used a high-resolution microscope to monitor the regenerative activity of scar tissue in a heart damaged by a heart attack. He

---

[30] Warner, Jennifer, "Brain May Suffer Long After Heart Bypass," *WebMD Medical News*, July 15, 2002, http://my.webmd.com/content/article1675.62736.

reported evidence of cell growth, although not sufficient to restore function in the damaged area. These findings will open new avenues of research into treatments for diseased hearts.

Mechanical Heart in the News

When I first wrote about the development of *cardiac assist devices*, I was aware that they were going into clinical trials. According to the manufacturer, the goal was to extend a patient's life during the time awaiting a heart transplant. We now know the outcome of those trials—at least the first phase. The "self-contained mechanical heart" kept a patient alive for about five months, longer than the manufacturer had anticipated. Naturally, this kind of news triggers lots of questions in people's minds. Listeners in my Sunday afternoon radio audience called and wanted more detail and my commentary on this development. If you read the news reports thoroughly, you will understand that the technology is in a very early experimental stage. The FDA allowed the manufacturer only five human patients in five different medical centers for the trials. The first reported took place in Lexington, KY. The patient was near death from heart disease and the procedure was expected to give him only several additional months to live.

How optimistic should we be about technology like this? Patients ask whether it would be available for them if they should need it. By the estimates of everyone involved, the doctors, the manufacturer, and government agencies that fund the research, the day when a mechanical heart will be a widespread practical therapy is not in sight. What is encouraging, however, is the pace and inventiveness of medical technology in the United States. Every year there is some new and beneficial technique or pharmaceutical available to us that is indeed lifesaving and can be used in practice immediately. It is for this reason that I motivate my patients and my radio audience to stay in good health so that they might live to benefit from the coming health care advances.

Artificial Heart Going into Trials

You never know what you might find searching "heart" categories on the Internet. On the website www.biomed.com, there's a picture of a beating heart on the home page of Abiomed,[31] a company that develops heart replacement products. A 5-minute video, which you can click to, describes the function of the Abiomed BVS 5000, an inplanted cardio assist

---

[31] Abiomed Inc., Danvers MA, www.biomed.com.

device currently used widely to take over the function of a failing heart. Their newer AbioCor, a heart replacement device, aims at permanently replacing heart transplants. It is said to allow users to functional normally and even participate in some light sports. The first experimental subjects will be five patients too sick for heart transplants. Costs are estimated from $75,000 to $100,000 per unit, relatively equal to the cost of coronary bypass surgery. The press notice in which this news was presented reported that there are 100,000 citizens with heart failure each year, but only 2,000 hearts available for transplant. Abiomed states its goals as "working toward the day when cessation of heart function will no longer be the end of life."

All of the subjects discussed in this section were developed from health news that is available in newspapers, periodicals, and now on the Internet. It is the grave responsibility of all health care practitioners to keep abreast of the news in health care science. Health information, today so easily available, works in two ways: it assists you with practical advice on how to maintain your personal health, and it motivates you in your resolve to advance toward the cure for heart disease.

Chapter Four

Miscellaneous Advice

Are You Following Your Doctor's Orders and Taking Your Medications?

"Your health is in your own hands" has been a slogan of mine throughout my practice. At no time is it more important than in following up your doctor's visit with strict attention to the directives you have received. After all, to what advantage are all the advances made in developing effective drugs—and they truly are marvelous—if patients neglect to take them?

Would you believe that 50 percent of patients are not following doctor's orders? In a review of various and varied surveys of patients' adherence in taking their prescriptions, researchers expressed alarm at what the data shows.[32] The surveys dealt with hypolipidemic drugs—the drugs prescribed for lowering cholesterol and lipids or fatty substances in the blood in general. Even in controlled clinical trials, in which subjects were carefully directed to follow the medication schedule and are supported throughout the trial period, adherence was surprisingly poor. In what the researchers call free-living populations (people not participating in clinical trials), the adherence is even poorer. For example, where adherence was measured by examining discontinuation rates in pharmacy dispensing databases, one report showed that "75 percent of new recipients of hypolipidemic agents had discontinued treatment at one year (defined as not obtaining a prescription refill for 90 days or more)."

There are different forms of nonadherence: some patients never get the prescription filled to begin with or don't get the prescription refilled; some take the wrong dosage or take the medication at the wrong time; some simply cease taking their medications altogether. What is particularly significant and regrettable about this nonadherence or noncompliance

---

[32] Tsuyuki, Ross T., et al., "Poor Adherence with Hypolipodic Drugs," [Pharmacotherapy], See Medscape www.medscape.com/viewarticle/40975.

is that there is so much evidence proving the efficacy of lipid-lowering drugs and their ability to counter the lethal effects of cardiovascular disease. A statin drug, such as Lipitor, is said to reduce cholesterol by 30-40 percent in less than a year's time and to lower the risk of heart attack by the same percentage.

The reasons for nonadherence are not as easily established by statistical study. However, the researchers offer some hypotheses. A number of factors influence nonadherence. Chronic diseases like heart disease and hypertension are asymptotic. Patients don't feel any symptoms, as they might take an aspirin if they felt a headache coming on. Moreover, the benefits of this therapy are preventive, avoiding a future adverse event that is not tangible. As a matter of fact, patients who have suffered a heart attack or stroke are found to be measurably more compliant in a secondary prevention program.

The elderly may have problems with adherence because of cognitive difficulties and complex drug regimens. Forgetfulness is the most commonly reported reason for nonadherence. If they are taking more than two drugs, seeing several physicians, and using two or more pharmacies, adherence is very likely to be poor. Education and cost may also influence nonadherence. There is slightly greater adherence among those with high school education. While cost could be a factor, there happens to be evidence of nonadherence among patients whose insurance covers drug costs.

Linking Peace of Mind to Good Health

We've known for a long time through research that depression is associated with heart disease. Depressed persons have an increased risk of heart attack—as much as double the risk of persons not suffering depression. Depression also increases the mortality rate of heart disease. One reason for depressed persons being more likely to have a heart attack or stroke, is that depression amplifies the effects of common risk factors. It does this by increasing athrosclerosis, the buildup of fatty deposits in the arteries. In one study, depressed smokers had three times the amount of athrosclerosis as smokers who were not depressed. The impact of LDL cholesterol on athrosclerosis was nearly twice as great in depressed men.

It is therefore well worth it for the sake of one's health—heart health in particular, since heart disease is life-threatening—to protect yourself against depression with an exercise program. That's for starters. You should also be aware of circumstances which may trigger depression: change in appetite resulting in unexpected weight loss. These include a change in sleeping patterns (sleeping too much or fitful sleep), loss of pleasure in activities formerly enjoyed, fatigue, feelings of worthlessness, inability to concentrate or make decisions, and overwhelming feelings of grief and sadness. Since depression can sometimes go unrecognized in a person, it's best to keep up an antidepression exercise program to be certain to be free of it.

How much is diet and exercise a factor in a positive mental attitude and fending off depression? A cluster of studies reported in the past year that assessed the effects of exercise and diet on mental health came up with the same conclusion.[33] A study involving more than 3,000 adults in Finland noted that those who ate fish frequently were less likely to suffer depression. It's a fact: fish is high in the polyunsaturated fatty acid Omega-3, a dietary supplement that has been used to treat depression. In two studies of exercise and depression among elderly subjects, researchers concluded that an age-related decrease in the intensity of physical exercise increases the risk of depressive symptoms. Unfortunately, as people age they are less physically able to exercise and even slow down all physical activity. The result is the depression that often accompanies advanced age; all the more reason why persons should deliberately adopt an exercise routine as they grown older. Stiffness, frailty, and decreased stamina should not be accepted deterrents, but should be overcome.

In another eleven-year long survey among seniors, the "mood-boosting power" of exercise was established. In fact, it was evident in the study that whenever people quit or fell off in their exercise activities, depression was likely to set in. To continue this line of inquiry, researchers at the University of Texas established a connection between positive mental attitude and good health. Emotional well-being was a strong predictor of the health status of subjects in this study of 200 men and women over 65. The link between happiness and good health held even after the researchers factored in chronic disease, smoking and drinking habits, and education.

If you haven't been on an exercise program and intend to start one in order to fend off depression, take note of a recent study from Duke University Medical Center. It found that a brisk 30-minute walk or jog three times a week will help to alleviate even major depressive disorders. After 16 weeks on an exercise program, patients in this study not only experienced the same relief from depression as a matched group on medication; they also felt more self-confident and had better self-esteem. But be

---

[33] O'Brien, Kelly, "Exercise for Mental Health," *Think Muscle Newsletter*, www.thinkmuscle.com/articles/obrien/exercise-for-mental-health.htm.

warned that you have to get into the program and stick with it in order to feel its benefits.

Alcohol and Your Heart

The subject of alcohol consumption and heart health regularly appears in the medical journals.[34] I have discussed this subject often in my newsletters over the years. The conclusions don't change much, but there is always value in examining the latest findings and looking at the characteristics of the data. In one study, researchers in Boston interviewed 1913 hospitalized heart attack victims, men and women, over a period of five years in the 1990s. Those who had seven or fewer drinks a week (light drinkers) were 20 percent less likely to die; and those who had seven or more drinks a week (moderate drinkers) were 30 percent less likely to die. There were no significant differences reflected in the data for the kind of drinks consumed—beer, wine, or whisky. Another study reported similar results: moderate drinkers (1-1½ drinks a day) were 20 percent to nearly 50 percent less likely to develop heart failure than nondrinkers. These findings are clear on the relationship of drinking to heart disease to the extent that the design of the research could determine. In practice, however, there are always variables to be aware of when advising individual patients.

When Maria Santoro, the nutritionist in my practice, and I researched this subject for my newsletters, we noted that alcohol works in a couple of ways that are beneficial to the heart. It raises HDL, the good cholesterol. It also protects against the formation of dangerous blood clots that lead to heart attacks, by raising the level of the naturally occurring enzyme *tissue-type plasminogen activator,* or TPA. Highest levels of TPA have been found in moderate drinkers and lowest levels among nondrinkers.

But since we are always concerned about our patients' overweight condition, we have to warn that alcohol adds calories and may also increase triglycerides (that's fat) in the blood, thus adding risks from another direction. We are also reminded of these statistics: the habit of more than three drinks a day is related to increased mortality; and an estimated 100,000 deaths annually, which could be avoided, are attributed to alcohol related causes. It is obvious, therefore, that alcohol's benefits for heart

---

[34] Abramson, Jerome L., et al., "Moderate Alcohol Consumption and Risk of Heart Failure Among Older Persons," *JAMA,* April 18, 2001.

health notwithstanding, there will be no public health recommendations advocating alcohol consumption. As a practical guide, we have put together a set of principles by which to judge the appropriate use of drinking alcohol with respect to heart health:

- One to two drinks a day may have a beneficial effect. More than that is associated with increased health risks.
- Persons at risk for alcohol addiction because of prior addiction or family history should avoid all alcohol beverages.
- Even moderate alcohol consumption should not occur at times when work, operating a motor vehicle, or other functions will be impaired.
- People with certain health problems should avoid alcohol altogether. These include liver disease, congestive heart failure, and degenerative neurological conditions, to mention a few.

And if you are really serious about your heart health, you should make sure you discuss your use of alcohol with your doctor.

New Classifications of Heart Failure

When the doctor examining you asks if you have any shortness of breath or swelling of your ankles, when he (or she) places the stethoscope on your chest and back and asks you to breath normally, he is trying to determine whether you have any symptoms of heart failure. Three million Americans suffer this condition. It is defined as an inability of the mechanism of the heart to pump enough blood to supply the other parts of the body. Pretty basic. And when the condition is acute, it is extremely life threatening. But there are different stages of heart failure; and by taking note of them medical experts believe that heart failure is treatable and will respond beneficially to specific therapies.

In November 2001, the American Heart Association, jointly with the American College of Cardiology, announced new definitions of the stages of heart failure.[35] These new stages or classifications are intended to guide physicians in the treatment of heart failure that takes advantage of the most recent scientific and pharmaceutical advances.

---

[35] "Practice Guidelines," *Circulation,* Journal of the American Heart Association, December 11, 2001, www.acc.org.

Stage A: Patients have no symptoms and no damage to their heart; but they have risk factors, like family history, overweight, diabetes, high blood pressure.

Stage B: Patients have no symptoms but have some damage of their heart muscle, either from a disease or heart attack or a congenital condition.

Stage C: Patients have damage <u>and</u> symptoms. In a heart attack or *myocardium infarction,* arteries in the heart burst and permanently disable areas of heart muscle. It is believed heart muscle, once damaged in this can never recover to function again.

Stage D: Patients with acute heart failure, which require hospitalization.

Among the modern drugs used to treat heart failure, particularly in pre-acute stages, is the ACE inhibitor. It is manufactured by at least 10 pharmaceutical companies. Recent and ongoing clinical trials of the ACE inhibitor *ramipril* (brand name Altace) have established some remarkable results in the treatment of hypertension and heart diseases. ACE stands for Angiotensin Converting Enzyme. Angiotensin is a neurohormone, which in a converted form affects blood vessels by making them shrink. When it is inhibited by the presence of the drug, blood vessels will remain supple, less constricted. It should be obvious why a drug that affects our blood vessels in a positive way is a therapy for hypertension. Taken a step further, by easing the flow of blood in the heart, it eases the heart's pumping work and, in fact, has been shown to reverse the effect of heart failure and restore the heart to its normal pumping function.

ACE inhibitor drugs are recommended therapy not only when heart failure is in stages B and C, but also as a preventive therapy when there are no symptoms of heart failure but only the risks (stages A and B). Recent studies have also pointed to the importance of adequate dosages of the ACE inhibitor, in order to benefit from its effect. When there are reports of side effects, which some patients cannot tolerate, one solution is changing to another brand. A safe and effective dosage might be that administered in the HOPE study which demonstrated the benefits of *ramipril* —20mg. Altace, the brand name for ramipril, is a very highly promoted drug these days. Your doctor may have some samples in his office. Ask him about it.

Heart Attack Diagnosis in the ER

When a person comes to a hospital emergency room complaining of chest pain, what can be expected? If he or she is diagnosed immediately as having heart disease or having a heart attack, what effect will that have on the long term outcome? Put in simpler terms, if they have a heart-attack and are treated for it are their chances of survival better? Of course the answer is *yes*. But, there is plenty more to be learned about chest pain and its treatment, about the risk factors for heart disease, and about ER diagnosis. Scientists in Sweden have been investigating these questions for ten years or more. They published the findings of their latest study in the *American Heart Journal*.[36] In following up on 5,362 patients who had come into a hospital ER with chest pain or other indicators of possible heart attack (acute coronary infarction or ACI), the authors came to certain conclusions that can be used in assessing your own heart health situation and fostering a preventive attitude. Over the ten-year period, 29 percent of the patients died, virtually all of heart related causes.

- The older the patient, the greater the mortality risk.
- Men are at greater risk than women, probably because more heart disease is found in men than in women.
- A history of diabetes mellitus increased the risk of death about 80 percent.
- A history of smoking increased the risk of death less than 50 percent. But the researchers note the complexity of measuring this factor, since patients with other risk factors, such as diabetes, hypertension, and previous heart attack are likely to have become nonsmokers. The study strongly supports "the importance of anti-smoking advice."
- Having had a heart attack previously is also an indicator of an adverse outcome, especially for older persons.
- Absence of chest pain when other indicators of heart disease are present is an "unfavorable sign" that may be related to congestive heart failure.

---

[36] Herlitz, Johan, et al., "Important factors for the 10-year mortality rate in patients with acute chest pain or other symptoms consistent with acute myocardial infarction with particular emphasis on the influence of age," *American Heart Journal*, October 2001.

These findings are not in themselves surprising. What the study's authors point out is that for the purpose of diagnosis, when a patient comes to the ER with acute chest pain or other symptoms consistent with heart attack, the patients' risk factors and past history are more likely to influence the outcome the younger (under 65) the patient is.

Sex After 60 Is Better Than in Middle Age

Most Americans over age 60 who have responded to a recent survey about their sexual activity reported that their sex life in their sixties and seventies is actually more fulfilling than it was in middle age. Women were more likely to be emotionally satisfied compared with men: 65 percent versus 42 percent. Among the reasons given for increased satisfaction was a new marriage or relationship, being more in touch with each other, no children to disturb them, more time to enjoy sex, and less stress. Some 26 percent say that sex was less satisfying than it used to be, and more than half of this group attributed the decline to a medical condition or to the natural aging process. The sponsor of the survey, Pfizer Pharmaceutical, manufacturers of *Viagra*, suggests the problem of less satisfying sex whether caused by a medical condition or aging, is "fixable".[37]

Lifestyle that Promotes Heart Health Also Assists Male Sexual Function

Cardiovascular problems and male sexual dysfunction are often connected. Risk factors for heart disease are also risk factors for impotence. For instance, a low level of HDL cholesterol (the good cholesterol), which is a risk factor for heart disease, also has been found to be significantly correlated with sexual dysfunction in men. Smoking and heart disease are especially predictive of impotence. Impotence also can be a symptom of disease. And, of course, medications used to treat high blood pressure may often cause sexual dysfunction.

Sexual dysfunction, which means loss of desire as well as difficulties of performance, can be the result of problems in a relationship. But, physical causes often exist for sexual dysfunction. In dealing with sexual difficulties, it's important to evaluate your general health. Being overweight and inactive can contribute significantly. Alcohol, marijuana, and

---

[37] Pfizer Global Study of Sexual Attitudes and Behavior (an ongoing study), www.pfizerglobalstudy.com

cocaine, often used by people as sexual stimulants, are actually sexual depressants. Those lifestyle changes that promote a healthy heart also promote healthy sexual functioning, and behavioral modifications should be tried before any other therapy. I suggest some rules to follow:

1. Not more than one drink a day.
2. No recreational drugs.
3. Regular exercise.
4. Maintain appropriate weight.

There are a number of other steps you can take as well.

- *Check your blood pressure medication.* Beta-blockers and diuretics, prescribed for high blood pressure, are notorious for causing impotence. Other medications will help your blood pressure without this side effect. Ask your doctor about switching to an alpha-blocker or an ACE inhibitor. They do not seem to affect sexual functioning.
- *Have your diabetic status evaluated.* Diabetes causes a high rate of sexual dysfunction.
- *Ask your physician about aorta iliac duplex imaging.* This is a way to check large blood vessels in the stomach that supply the penis with blood, which enables you to get and maintain an erection.
- *Have your testosterone measured.* The normal range is 200 to 1000. If you are on the low side, you may want to consider supplementation. Use natural testosterone, available in compounding pharmacies.
- *Have your vitamin status checked and replace deficiencies.* Vitamins that help impotence include: a general antioxidant formula, zinc, argenine (for sperm development), and extra vitamin B-5 for adrenal support. Yohimbine, an herb from the bark of a tree, has been shown to improve erectile function. (Caution: It may cause arrhythmia.) It is available at some health food stores and by prescription.

This raises the question: Is there a male menopause? While we acknowledge that women experience a hormone decline with age and often require or desire estrogen replacement, we have not fully investigated the similar decline in men. We know that testosterone decreases with age, as does DHEA, a hormone produced by the adrenals. This decline in hormones is associated with increased cardiovascular disease, arteriosclerosis, loss of muscle development, and sexual dysfunction. Preliminary but promising research is underway to investigate whether testosterone supplementation will alleviate these problems.

The normal range for testosterone is 200 to 1000. Men who measure on the low side, say around 300, may be told by their physicians that they are in the normal range. But, in fact, if testosterone supplementation is used to bring the patient up to the high end of that range, sexual performance may be enhanced. Testosterone can be taken by injection or orally. A caveat: If you have prostate cancer, testosterone can accelerate its growth. Before prescribing testosterone, I first do a prostate ultrasound and prostate-specific antigen (PSA), which tests for cancer. I monitor very carefully anyone on testosterone.

Sex After a Heart Attack

Questions of heart disease and intimacy are addressed in two recent books *Heart Illness and Intimacy* by Wayne Sotile Ph.D., and *Love and Survival: Eight Pathways to Intimacy and Health*, by Dean Ornish M.D., the renown pioneer of heart disease prevention.[38] What is needed most to ease people's anxieties in this area is information. Here are some solid facts gleaned from these two publications.

- The risk of a subsequent heart attack caused by sex is less than 1 percent, and regular exercise can lower that risk even more.
- The increased heart rate that accompanies sex is often only as strenuous as gardening or climbing a couple flights of stairs.
- Intimacy and sex have a positive effect on one's well-being and that is good for a healthy recovery.
- Viagra and other medications designed to boost sex drive are generally safe; however, they should only be used after a consult with a physician.

There are support groups for spouses that offer comfort to persons adjusting after a heart attack in the family. It might be a good idea to check your local hospital for a schedule of meetings.

---

[38] Sotile, Wayne, Ph.D., *Heart Illness and Intimacy*, Books on Demand, 1992; Ornish, Dean, M.D., *Love and Survival: Eight Pathways to Intimacy and Health*, Harper Perennial, NY, 1998.

A Men's Health Brief

A survey by the men's magazine *Men's Health*[39] has uncovered the rather unhealthy eating habits of the average American male. His favorite snack is potato chips, and the meal he is most likely to prepare for a romantic date is spaghetti. The survey (not claiming to be scientific) also revealed that the odds that a man will eat fast food on any given day is 1 in 2.5. The average male consumes 26 pounds of beef, 57 pounds of chicken, 16 pounds of cheese, 17 pounds of fish, 11 pounds of pork, 19 pizza pies, and 603 cups of coffee each year. All this adds up to an average annual weight gain of 1.1 pounds. Dr Chris Rosenbloom, a spokesperson for the American Dietetic Association, said the survey demonstrated the attitude of the average male is "I want the body that is on the cover of *Men's Health*, but I don't want to eat well to get there." For the record, among the groups contacted for the survey were the Texas Department of Corrections and the Snack Food Association. Not that women are any more consistent in their dietary habits, at least as inferred from their popular magazines. Says Dr. Rosenbloom, "I see gorgeous women on the covers and then I see 30 recipes for cookies inside."

---

[39] "The Average Guy," *Men's Health*, April 2001, www.menshealth.com.

Chapter Five

Maria Santoro's Healthy Kitchen

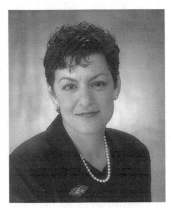

Introducing Maria Santoro, R.D.

Maria Santoro has worked with me for almost a decade. She is a Registered Dietician and a nutrition specialist. Each month she contributed a piece to the *Wellness Newsletter* on a topic that was based on her daily clinical work. As you will see in the following pages, her commentary is very practical: she gives suggestions on how to shop when you are trying to control your weight, or what kind of foods you can include in your smart eating program that will make your meals exciting. Patients who need to manage their food intake in order to protect their health are directed to sit down with Maria. Her interviews are insightful; she directs patients with great confidence and inspires them to keep up their health diet discipline. That is what accounts for her success. You will have that experience as you read on.

Dieting Techniques

When patients come to the office for help in losing weight, I provide them with a number of techniques for success. I assist them in making the behavioral changes that will lead to achieving their desired goals.

For example, I always try to get patients to verbalize their "weak links" with regard to eating. What has kept them from losing weight in the past? For some people, it is stuffing food in their mouths, even when they're not hungry. These patients need to distinguish between eating because of stress or boredom and eating because of true hunger. Other patients don't plan their meals and as a result they don't have the right food in the house. This can result in eating the wrong thing because it's in the refrigerator, or picking up pizza on the way home from work.

Sometimes patients try to put themselves on an unreasonable diet, such as only oatmeal for breakfast and only tuna fish for lunch. In addition to being unhealthy, this kind of diet is doomed to failure because the body will crave the variety of foods that it needs. For many patients, the problem is that they don't know what to eat. They're not sure which foods have a high fat or calorie content. They may not be aware of healthy ways of cooking. They need to educate themselves. I give them menus and instruct them about reading food labels, cooking techniques, and meal planning.

On the other hand, some patients know perfectly well what they should do, but they don't do it. They need to set both short-term and long-term goals, and these goals must be both specific and attainable. Going on a diet because you want to look like Cindy Crawford is not a specific and attainable goal. Examples of appropriate long-term goals are: "I want to lose 30 pounds in six months," or "I want to drop enough weight by the end of the year to get off blood pressure medication."

Short-term goals are also introduced—no more than one or two a week—to put the patient on the path toward the long-term goal. For example, appropriate goals would be: "I will exercise three times a week at the gym for 45 minutes" or, "I will not go to a fast food restaurant more than once a week." Patients tend to set unrealistic goals, such as "Ill never eat fast food again," or "I want to lose 15 pounds in a month," so I try to help them be more practical. It's important to make sure that patients are ready to add a new short-term goal and be comfortable with the level of the goal.

The Daily Practice of Dieting

At the Wellness Centers, we work with hundreds of patients who are trying to lose weight. Many of them come in because they want a magic bullet that will make the pounds melt away. While we don't have that kind of instant solution, we can provide them with help and useful advice. We try to get these patients to make small behavioral changes that will assist with their weight loss as outlined below.

- Make a plan to trim 200 to 300 calories from your diet each day.
- Have nutrition information readily available. You should own a calorie counter and carbohydrate gram counter to which you can refer when you're uncertain about the content of certain foods.
- Know what you are eating. Identify sources of hidden fat. Determine if you are consuming too much carbohydrate or protein. Read the labels on packaged food.
- Eat when you are reasonably hungry. You should time your meals and snacks to prevent extreme hunger. Eat slowly and savor your meals. You should take at least 20 minutes to eat a meal, and put down your fork at least three or four times.
- Fill up on high fiber foods, especially vegetables. Stop eating when you are comfortably full, not stuffed.
- Ride out cravings or satisfy them with small portions. Limit exposure to foods you crave—don't keep them in the house. Always have healthy foods available. Find nonfood substitutes, such as taking a walk or a soaking in a relaxing bath, to distract you from cravings.
- Shop wisely. Plan your meals for a week and prepare a shopping list. Buy only what is on the list. Don't shop on an empty stomach. Stay away from the supermarket deli counter—it's loaded with high-fat foods. Stock up on a lot of fresh greens.
- Avoid fad diets and extreme calorie restrictions. Make sure your eating plan allows room for your favorites occasionally.
- When setting your weight loss goals, be realistic about genetics and body type. Determine the weight you would like to achieve and set a reasonable time in which to reach your goal. Lose only one to two pounds a week.
- Maintain a food journal. Keep track of what you eat and the reasons you eat. Are you eating for reasons other than hunger, such as stress or boredom?
- Drink eight glasses of water a day. Don't substitute juice, soda, milk, or other beverages.
- Don't forget about exercise. You should have at least 20 minutes a day of reasonable vigorous exercise. If you don't want to join a gym, take a brisk walk or use an exercise bicycle while watching TV or videos.

The Fruit and Vegetable Rule

Most people should have five to nine servings of fruit and vegetables a day in order to achieve good health. (There is an exception to this rule: Those with insulin resistance and diabetes must limit their consumption of fruit on an individualized basis.) Americans on average consume no more than two or three servings of fruit and vegetables per day. People give a number of reasons why they find it difficult to eat enough fruit and vegetables. They may believe that vegetables take too long to prepare or that produce spoils too quickly and therefore is not at hand when needed. Some people just don't like fruit and vegetables. And, let's face it: out-of-season fruit and vegetables often don't taste very good. If these are your objections, here are some tips to help you get your daily supply:

- Find a good produce store or go to a farmer's market. The fresher fruit and vegetables are, the better they taste. Fresh asparagus right off the farm, for instance, is vastly superior to the canned or frozen variety.
- Having said that, however, also remember not to be a fresh produce snob. While fresh is best, it's not always the most convenient. Don't sneer at frozen or canned fruit and vegetables. They may not taste as good as fresh, but generally they have comparable nutritional benefits and should be used if fresh ones are not available. (Frozen is better than canned, which often have excess sodium.)
- Buy bagged salad greens if you don't want to take the time to clean and prepare lettuce. Don't use the dressings that come with the bagged greens, however, since they tend to be high in fat and calories. Make your own light oil and lemon dressing and keep it in the refrigerator or buy a low-calorie bottled dressing.
- Keep several days worth of salad greens in the salad spinner.
- Buy the "grape" tomatoes now available in most supermarkets. Unlike regular tomatoes, they are sweet and tasty all year round and they can be added to a salad without even the effort of slicing.
- Buy cleaned and packaged celery sticks, broccoli, and carrots to use as snacks. Buy packaged, grated cabbage to use for coleslaw.
- Keep a bowl of washed fresh fruit on the table for snacking.
- If you're really rushed, use the salad bar in the supermarket.
- It's not very difficult to cut up a head of broccoli, steam it, and add lemon juice, or put a whole acorn squash in the microwave for 10 minutes and bake it. Cooking doesn't get much easier than that.

- If you have insulin resistance or diabetes, discuss your fruit intake with your physician.

Shopping Strategies

You must begin your battle against fat by becoming a supermarket warrior. If you buy only nourishing, healthy food, chances are that's what you will eat. Here's how to avoid stuffing your cupboards and refrigerators with foods that are not good for you.

- Plan your meals for the week. Prepare a shopping list and buy only what's on the list. This will keep you from impulse buying (and probably save you money and time as well).
- Shop the perimeters of the food market. That's where you'll find fresh vegetables and fruit, as well as fresh fish and unprocessed lean meats.
- Stock up on a lot of fresh greens.
- Know your supermarket layout. Do not go down the aisles containing sweets and snack food.
- Do not shop on an empty stomach. Have a piece of fruit, fresh veggies, or a glass of seltzer beforehand.
- Be careful in the frozen food aisle. It contains many breaded and high salt items.
- If you buy a whole roasted chicken, ask the deli person to take off the skin before it leaves the market.
- Inquire at the deli counter as to which foods are low fat and low salt.
- Don't be tempted by the prepared foods at the deli counter. They usually are fried or loaded with mayonnaise.
- Do not open and eat any food while shopping.
- If you are not used to label reading, prepare yourself for this before you go to the market; then take the time to read them. Be a detective.
- Remember that the ingredients on the label are listed from the largest to smallest quantity.
- The total fat per serving in the food you select should be less than three grams per 100 calories. The ratio of unsaturated to saturated fat should be two to one.

- Have no more than 300 mg of total cholesterol per day. If it comes from an animal, it has cholesterol.
- If the package says low fat, be sure to check the calories. A product can be very low in fat, yet high in calories. Experts believe that lack of awareness of this fact may be one of the main reasons that Americans are getting fatter.
- Watch the salt content on labels. You should have no more than 2000 mg per day.
- Select foods with no more than five grams of sugar per serving.

Eating on the Run

During my initial meeting with new patients, I ask them to describe their eating history and habits. (Anything they consume more than twice a week is considered a habit.) Getting this information has made me something of an expert on what people do wrong nutritionally and how they sabotage their efforts to lose weight and maintain health. Probably the biggest problem I see is that most people eat breakfast and lunch on the run. They never seem to actually sit down at a table for an unhurried meal. Their typical breakfast is a donut or a bagel with cream cheese, accompanied by coffee with cream and sugar and eaten in their car or at their desk. Even those who are making an effort to improve their diets are not doing much better. They may consume fat free muffins or a white roll, but usually it's slathered with butter. These are foods high in saturated fat, hydrogenated oil, and calories and low in fiber—a perfect recipe for weight gain and heart disease.

Over the last two years, a new breakfast problem has emerged—specialty coffee shops offering frappacino and cappucino. People mistakenly believe that these are low calorie treats. In fact, they usually contain sugary syrups, hydrogenated oil, and even heavy cream. Lunch on the run from the local deli or a fast food restaurant creates even more problems. Mayonnaise is rampant at lunchtime in macaroni or potato salad. If it's on a sandwich along with cold cuts such as bologna or cheese you have a lunch laden with unhealthy fats and calories. At fast food restaurants, chicken nuggets and cheeseburgers are favorites. Even people who decide to eat healthy and have a salad often ladle hundreds of fat-drenched calories in the form of dressing over the salad. The dressings at some of the fast food places have as much as 20 grams of fat.

Many patients want to do better, but they don't know what to order when they eat on the run. Sandwiches should be on enriched wheat or whole grain bread with mustard, not mayonnaise. Forget about hero rolls. Turkey, chicken, canned tuna, and alpine lace cheese are acceptable cold cuts. When you have coleslaw or cucumber and tomato salad, drain off the excess liquid. If you have a salad, ask for the low fat dressing on the side. Don't eat at your desk or in the car. Take a real break and get away from it all, perhaps to a park bench, even if it's for only 15 minutes.

Conquer Dietary Pitfalls

You come home from work late after a stressful day. You're exhausted. You're tense. You're hungry. The last thing you care about is preparing a healthy meal. You look in the refrigerator and shove into your mouth whatever is there, that requires the least effort to prepare. This sort of situation happens all too often. When you're in a less stressed-out mood a healthy eating program seems like an excellent idea. But then life gets complicated and it's just too much trouble. Here are tips to get you through those times.

When you get home from work, sit down in a comfortable chair. Take five or six long, deep breaths. Give yourself five to ten minutes before entering the kitchen. You probably are in a fog after a long day of work, especially if you have a long commute. Give yourself time to relax and to become aware of true physiological hunger. Plan your meals. Be aware of when your next meal will be. Have appropriate food in the refrigerator at all times. If the only thing in the refrigerator is cold pizza, that's probably what you will eat. Here are some more tips:

- Warm up your food. Warm foods have more flavor, thereby slowing down your eating by reaching the preferred taste quicker.
- When you are ready to eat, give yourself a limit and put only that amount on your plate. Pay attention to your food.
- Maximize satisfaction. Eat the foods you enjoy in moderation. Do not force yourself to eat a certain food because it is on your diet.
- Eliminate distractions. Focus on what you are eating. If there is noise or other distractions around you, stop eating for a moment, shut your eyes, take a deep breath, and relax.
- Chew every morsel of your food. Cut your food using a fork and knife.

- Watch your appetite change during a meal. The first bite tastes the best. If you are no longer hungry, and you are not savoring the food, that's the time to stop.
- Sit down during your meal. Standing over the kitchen counter is not relaxing and can promote overeating.
- Do not skip two meals consecutively. Hunger will build and eventually your eating will go out of control. For some people this happens if they skip even one meal.
- Listen to your sweet tooth. If you yearn for dessert, have a sensible treat within an hour after dinner.
- Make eating a pleasurable experience.

How to Survive the Holidays

I see many patients who gain as much as 5 to 15 pounds in the 40 days between Thanksgiving and New Year's Day. They regard the holidays as a license to eat, and they swear they'll get down to business and lose their new extra pounds in January. Food is a part of our holiday tradition, so people should be able to eat and enjoy themselves. At the same time, they must try to exercise some restraint. If you are on a diet, you don't have to lose weight during this time period, but you should strive to prevent that holiday bulge.

To avoid weight gain, it's important to have a blueprint for the entire holiday season. Think about all the parties, dinners, and other celebrations you will attend and have a strategy for enjoying them without "pigging out." Be flexible, sensible, and conscious of what you eat. You should organize food shopping so that you have plenty of healthy low-fat, low-calorie food to eat at home. You'll be busy, and you don't want to just "grab and go," eating whatever happens to be in the refrigerator or grabbing a bite at the mall.

Never go to a party hungry and don't skip meals so you can eat all you want at the event. Be sure to have a light breakfast, a light lunch, and then, before you leave, a snack of high-fiber cereal, salad, or vegetable soup. Drink plenty of water. When you get to the party, choose seltzer water or a diluted wine spritzer. Too much alcohol will lower your resistance to food and diminish your awareness of what you are eating. Don't gobble down food just because it's there. Don't stand around the food table. Put a little bit of everything you like on your plate, and then leave the area. Don't deprive yourself of your favorites; this leads to frustration and overeating, perhaps later when you get home. Engage in conversation.

You can't eat and talk at the same time. You may be surprised to learn you can enjoy a party even if you don't focus on food.

Unfortunately, many people become so busy with holiday activities that they give up their exercise programs and don't reestablish them until after the New Year. Even though time is scarce, it's important to take at least 20 to 30 minutes each day for an exercise activity as part of your blueprint for a healthy holiday.

How Garlic Lowers Lipids

If you are one of the people who believes there is no such thing as too much garlic, you are receiving some great health advantages. In addition to the taste benefits, garlic may help prevent heart disease. It benefits your health in a number of ways, most notably by lowering cholesterol. It aids in reducing blood pressure, lessens the tendency of the blood to form clots, and reduces stiffness of the arteries. Garlic is also reputed to strengthen the immune system and even to assist in the prevention of cancer. In numerous research studies, a daily dose of garlic—usually one half to one clove—has been demonstrated to reduce the cholesterol level between 15 and 20 percent. Garlic tablets also have a positive effect on cholesterol levels—but aren't nearly as enjoyable as real garlic.

There are many ways to use garlic in your cooking. It is most robust when it's raw, milder when quickly sautéed, and sweet when boiled or baked. Remember, however, that you want to eat the garlic itself, not just use it as a flavoring. For instance, garlic can be slow baked to produce a sweet nutty flavor and buttery consistency. Just place whole, unpeeled bulbs, round side down, in a shallow baking dish. Drizzle with a little oil, cover with foil and bake in a 325-degree oven for an hour and a half. The garlic juice can then be squeezed from the cloves and used as a low-fat spread on bread, added to a sauce, spread over grilled or roasted meat, or used in pasta sauces or salad dressings. When roasting beef, veal, or lamb, cut slits in the meat and insert slivers of garlic into each gash. The garlic will melt into the meat as it cooks. You can also roast whole garlic cloves along with the meat or poultry; then when it is done, take the garlic from the pan and purée it and add to the gravy.

You can sauté finely chopped garlic in a little olive oil and add it to cooked spinach, a pasta sauce, or a variety of other meat and vegetable dishes. Or you can use a little chopped raw garlic in salad dressing. When shopping for garlic, choose bulbs that are plump and compact, free of damp or soft spots. The outer skin should be taut and unbroken. It should feel heavy and firm in your hand; if it is light or gives under your finger, the contents may have dried out. Store garlic in a cool, dark spot in a loosely covered container.

Getting the Fat Out of Your Diet

Here are tips for controlling the amount of fat and cholesterol in your diet, particularly avoiding the saturated fats that are in meats and dairy products:

- Eat no more than six to eight ounces of meat, fish, or poultry each day. The meat should be lean, with all fat trimmed off before cooking. With poultry, remove skin as well as the fat under the skin before cooking. If you are roasting the bird, trim excess fat. To keep it from drying out, marinate it in chicken broth and baste often with the broth. Cover with aluminum foil during part of the roasting to keep it moist.
- Remember that some turkeys and chickens are injected with fat to keep them moist. Read the labels and avoid these.
- When buying ground beef, select the lean or extra lean. Buy "choice" or "select" grades of beef, rather than "prime." These are less expensive and also have less fat.
- Use cooking methods for meat, fish, and poultry that require little or no fat: boil, broil, bake, roast, poach, steam, sauté, stir-fry, or microwave. To enhance flavor use a little olive oil, lemon, wine, or just plain water.
- Avoid organ meats, such as sweetbreads, liver, or chitterlings, because they are very high in cholesterol.
- Limit yourself to three to four egg yolks a week. They are high in cholesterol. You may eat unlimited egg whites or egg substitutes, such as Eggbeaters.
- Always choose skim milk or one percent milk. These provide the same nutrients as whole milk, but without the fat, cholesterol, and calories. Avoid two percent milk as it is high in fat. If you don't like the taste of skim or one percent milk, make the changeover gradually. Try two percent milk, and then over time gradually mix in larger amounts of skim milk. Or, the taste of skim or one percent milk can be enhanced with unsweetened cocoa or other low-fat drink powders. You may also use milk from nonfat or low-fat

powder, evaporated skim milk, and buttermilk made from skim or one percent milk.

- Use low fat cheeses (less than three grams of fat per ounce). Dry curd or low fat cottage cheese is a good selection.
- The beginning of a new year (or month, or day) is a great time to focus on the importance of total health. Make time each day to incorporate exercise into your schedule—just do it. Once the sneakers are on, it easy to get going. Focus on the way you want your body to look. Start and end each day by focusing on your ultimate goals.

Potassium in Your Diet

If you have high blood pressure, cutting back on sodium is not enough. You should be sure you are getting enough potassium in your diet as well. These two minerals are linked and you must adjust your intake of both of them in order to get control of your blood pressure.

Not only does potassium help to regulate blood pressure, it has been shown to prevent strokes. In a study that tracked 44,000 men for eight years,[40] it was discovered that those people whose diet included large amounts of potassium had one-third fewer strokes, and the benefits were greatest for those with high blood pressure. The hypertensive men who took potassium supplements of one gram a day had a 60 percent lower risk of stroke than those with high blood pressure who did not take potassium supplements.

I see many people who are careful about their diets, and they believe they get enough potassium without supplements. I remind them, however, that certain conditions deplete the body's potassium and a greater intake is needed. If you are taking diuretics, which are frequently prescribed to control high blood pressure, the increased urinary loss that results will cause you to excrete more potassium. Other medications that deplete our stores of potassium include cortisone and prolonged use of aspirin and laxatives. Any fluid loss, sweating, vomiting, or diarrhea can also cause potassium loss, as can very low calorie diets. Symptoms of potassium depletion include extreme fatigue, muscle weakness, dry skin, and mental confusion.

---

[40] *Study: Potassium helps reduce blood pressure*, CNN/Health Story page, May 27, 1997, http://www.cnn.com/HEALTH/9705/27/potassium.bp/.

You need about 2 to 2.5 grams (2000 to 2500 mg) of potassium a day, but if you have a condition that is depleting potassium, you may need more. Your doctor can measure your potassium level with a simple blood test. He may suggest improving your diet or he may prescribe a potassium supplement. You should not take a potassium supplement unless you have checked with your doctor. Here are some foods high in potassium that can easily be incorporated into your diet:

- Peanuts (2 1/2 oz), 740 mg
- Cooked white beans (1/2 cup), 416 mg
- Banana (1 medium), 569 mg
- Carrots (2 small), 341 mg
- Chicken (light meat, 3 oz), 350 mg

*Other good sources include fish, especially salmon, flounder, cod, sardines, and leafy green vegetables.

Put Some Sizzle in Your Life

Grilling outdoors on the deck or patio doesn't have to be the ruin of your healthy eating habits. Forget hamburgers and hot dogs. This is an opportunity for culinary adventure, because grilling is an easy way to cook up first-rate, low-fat food.

- Use lean meat, such as skinless chicken breast, pork loin chops, lean cuts of beef, such as eye of round, and fish. Cut off any visible fat. Grilling will allow the remaining fat to drip away.
- Fish that grills well includes firm-textured fish such as tuna, swordfish, and mahi mahi, as well as scallops and shrimp.
- Use marinades and rubs. Marinades can be made with a variety of no-fat or low-fat ingredients such as wine, vinegar, lemon juice, yogurt, with seasonings added. Choose a marinade that does not include sugar or a sweet ingredient such as honey because it may blacken too much on the grill. Rubs are blends of dry herbs and spices that are worked into the meat to give it flavor. Experiment with your favorite seasonings such as rosemary, thyme, or oregano.
- For an even more interesting flavor, use one of the wide variety of wood chips available, such as mesquite or hickory.
- Don't forget about vegetables. For example, slice or chop green peppers, eggplant, and zucchini, with basil, parsley, onion, and garlic. Wrap them in aluminum foil coated with cooking spray and grill for 10 or 15 minutes. Or make up your own combinations.

- Try foil cookery for meat or fish too. Use heavy-duty foil and seal it tight to keep in the juices. Use fresh herbs generously. Combine fish, lemon, onion, dill, and parsley.
- Small cuts of meat, such as thin chops or cubed meat for kabobs, can be cooked directly over the coals. Larger cuts should be cooked over indirect heat. Bank the coals around the edges of the grate and put a drip pan in the middle. Then place the meat on the grill over the pan, cover, and roast.
- Perfect your timing. Grilling outdoors is trickier than cooking on a stove because you have less control of the heat. You don't want dried out, overcooked chops or dangerously undercooked chicken. Turkey burgers will be done in about 10 minutes. Chicken breasts and fish steaks should be ready in 15 minutes or less. To test for doneness, be sure that meat and poultry juices run clear and that fish flakes easily.
- If grilling over charcoal, wait until the coals are ash-colored and glowing. If using a gas or electric grill, ignite and cover for 5 to 10 minutes before starting to grill.

Spicing Up the Diet

With a little inventiveness, you can have tasty and satisfying meals while on The Wellness Centers' *Insulin-Regulating Diet.* There is no need for your food to be boring and bland. Here are some tips for making meals taste good, as well as hints for saving time when cooking and shopping.

- Chicken can be poached, steamed, or broiled. You can add lemon or lime or a little wine and any dried or fresh herbs. Poach chicken in a broth. If cooking on a grill, put the chicken in aluminum foil and add broth or wine. You can even add vegetables: peppers and tomatoes, for example. If you are in a hurry, you can purchase a whole roasted chicken at the supermarket, but remove all the skin and fat. Or you can buy sliced roasted chicken breast or roasted turkey breast (smoked, honey roasted, or peppered are all OK) at the deli counter.
- Fish can be prepared in the same manner as chicken: poached, steamed or grilled. Any of a wide variety of fish may be selected: tuna, flounder, sea bass, swordfish, clams, and salmon. Use dill, cilantro, parsley, basil, tarragon, or other fresh or dried herbs. If you are in a hurry, consider canned salmon or tuna packed in water.

- Vegetables can be fresh, canned (with no salt added or with salt rinsed off), or frozen (without the seasoning packet). You can add lemon and herbs to the vegetables.
- Fresh prepackaged vegetables, such as carrots and celery, will be of help to those in a hurry. Prepackaged salad greens, which should be washed, can be used, but skip the salad dressing mix that sometimes comes with the greens. It tends to be high in calories and salt.
- Vegetables you should not eat are: beets, peas, corn, potatoes, and yams. Also, do not eat legumes, such as lentils, kidney beans, lima beans, or black-eyed peas. These are all high in carbohydrates.
- If you want sauces to spice things up, try store-bought chili sauce, picante sauce or salsa, steak sauce, tomato sauce, tomato paste, or hot pepper sauce.
- Allowed condiments on the diet are horseradish, ketchup, mustard (any except Dijonnaise), and relish.
- Instead of olive oil and vinegar on the salad, you may use prepared salad dressings that are fat free and contain less than 360 mg per two tablespoons.
- You may substitute a pear or grapefruit for the apple on the diet, if you wish. Do not substitute any other fruit.

Food Sensitivity

Many patients have come to me in my practice complaining of symptoms such as fatigue or "just not feeling well." They may not suspect that a food sensitivity or an allergy is the cause of their problem. With an allergy, a particular food triggers the immune system and a reaction occurs, usually within 15 to 30 minutes. Symptoms can range from hives to vomiting and diarrhea to the lethal anaphylactic shock. The person can usually immediately identify the food that caused the reaction. A food sensitivity, however, involves a delayed reaction and individuals may not recognize that it is related to what they have eaten. They may get a headache a few hours later or experience debilitating fatigue the next day. This reaction may be caused by a food or a food additive, such as the MSG used in Chinese food or the artificial coloring in processed foods. Ironically, individuals often have cravings for the food to which they are most sensitive.

Food allergy and sensitivity should not be confused with food intolerance, which is caused by the lack of an enzyme needed to digest that particular food. The most common are lactose intolerance, the inability to digest dairy products; and gluten intolerance, an inability to digest the protein in wheat and other grains. Sensitivities and intolerances are similar in that they are both abnormal physical responses to food, but they do not involve the immune system. They usually are more difficult to diagnose than allergies. To treat these conditions, we first identify the food that causes the reaction. Tests can help make this determination, but the best method is for the patient to keep a log of foods eaten and symptoms experienced. We then put the patient on an elimination/rotation diet, whereby the suspected foods are eliminated for one to two weeks, then slowly reintroduced under medical supervision.

Patients often say to me, "But I've eaten shrimp all my life. Why am I having this reaction now?" When the body is compromised by stress, lack of sleep, excessive intake of processed or refined foods, hormonal changes, or even inactivity, the immune system may be weakened and food reactions are more likely to appear. So, in addition to treating the condition, a counter program must also focus on rebuilding the immune system.

Ever Consider Strength Training?

At the Wellness Center, we always emphasize that both strength training and aerobic exercise are necessary in order to lose weight, attain general fitness, and control and improve chronic health conditions such as heart disease, diabetes, hypertension, osteoporosis, arthritis, and a host of other diseases and conditions. Strength training not only improves strength, it also helps increase metabolism by developing lean muscle mass. People lose about one-half pound of muscle each year after age 20. Unfortunately, for every pound of muscle you lose, your body will burn 50 fewer calories per day, making it much easier to put on extra pounds as you get older.

Adding strength training to your schedule will help delay the natural loss of muscle associated with aging. It also helps to improve insulin resistance, increase bone density, raise HDL cholesterol, and improve flexibility and posture. As little as 20 minutes twice a week of well-planned strength training exercise can bring about these improvements. Strength training can be performed at home with weights. If you do not know how to do strength-training exercises, find a professional at your local fitness center who will help you get started. Select eight to ten exercises that prioritize major muscle groups. Remember to do a minimum of one set of 8 to 12 repetitions for each muscle group. Use enough weight to fatigue your muscles by the last few repetitions. Keep the speed of your movements slow to moderate in performing each exercise.

In addition to strength training, we recommend aerobic exercise for all our patients. It helps to increase aerobic capacity, strengthen the heart, and decrease blood pressure, just to mention a few of its benefits. Aerobic exercise is also an essential part of any weight loss program. Aerobic exercise includes those activities that utilize large muscle groups in a continuous rhythmic motion, such as running, walking, dancing, jumping rope, and swimming. Twenty minutes of continuous aerobic exercise three times a week will significantly improve endurance and health. Of course, more is better.

Refining Your Exercise Program

When doing aerobic exercise be sure you understand how to find your target heart zone in order to get the most out of your exercise program. You want to challenge yourself (a brisk walk, not a leisurely stroll), but not overdo it. Most of us are already overburdened with work and family responsibilities, and we feel we don't have the time or energy that an exercise program requires. But for the sake of your health, it's essential to make time. Patients sometimes report that even though they conscientiously diet and exercise, they fail to lose weight or to get in shape. I encourage these patients to use a heart rate monitor to aid in achieving their fitness and weight loss goals. Using your heart rate as a guide when exercising can help you work out much more effectively.

Certain improvements in your fitness level are guaranteed to happen when you work out strenuously enough to elevate your heart rate to 50-100 percent of its maximum rate. (*Your maximum heart rate is established by subtracting your age from 220.*) This is the fastest your heart should beat. Whatever your objectives—cardiac rehabilitation, prevention of disease, weight management, or winning athletic competitions—you can achieve them by working out within certain target heart rate zones, which are represented as a percentage of your maximum heart rate. If you are working at 50-60 percent of your maximum heart rate, you are engaged in moderate activity. At 60-70 percent of your maximum heart rate, you are in the exercise zone for weight management. You will burn fat and calories effectively and you will lose weight. Aerobic training occurs at 70-80 percent of your maximum heart rate, and at this level you will improve your aerobic endurance and really strengthen your heart.

You can train within your target heart rate zone only if you know how fast your heart is beating during your workout. This can be determined with a heart rate monitor, which continuously tells you when you are in your target heart rate zone. A heart rate monitor can be purchased at many large sporting goods stores. Beginners should slowly build up to the higher part of their target zone. After six months or more of regular exercise, it's okay to hit 75 percent of your maximum heart rate; or, if you are in excellent physical condition even 80 percent. The gradual approach is especially important for the elderly.

It's possible to find your heart rate without a monitor. During exercise, stop and count your heart rate for ten seconds. Multiply that number by six to establish your working heart rate. Remember that before you engage in any exercise program you should consult your physician. Then, set your goals and reevaluate them continuously after they have been met. It is best to exercise five times a week. Your workout sessions can be as short as 20-30 minutes. Most important, however hectic your schedule, you must make a strong commitment to take time out to achieve fitness and good health.

Chapter Six
Nutrients

Nutrient supplements tend to be subjected to faddism; one is the latest fad for a while, then another. It all depends on how promotional media deals with them at any given time. In fact, natural substances which benefit our health have been around forever, and were not invented or discovered by health food enthusiasts. There is much known about the benefits of the popular nutrients, yet sometimes what scientists know about them gives rise to controversy. I am very much aware of the benefits of nutrients in my practice. I will recommend them to my patients when it is appropriate, just as I would drugs. But, mainly, I want my patients to be knowledgeable about nutrients and for that reason, in my health educational materials, I describe the most popular nutrients, their benefits, and where they may be obtained.

Calcium Builds Strong Bones
This mineral may also reduce blood pressure and help prevent colon cancer; a deficiency of it may cause rickets in children.

We think of calcium for promoting healthy bones and teeth and for preventing osteoporosis. And those are indeed very important functions performed by this mineral. The body also depends on calcium for heartbeat regulation, proper blood clotting, muscle contraction, the release of neurotransmitters, and many other tasks. When the level of calcium in the blood is too low to perform these jobs, calcium is taken from the bones to make up the difference, thus weakening them. A calcium deficiency in children can lead to rickets, which results in bone deformities; in adults, a low level of this mineral has been related to colon cancer.

Both men and women lose bone as they grow older, but after menopause women begin losing it more rapidly, and one in four of them develop osteoporosis, a weakening of the bones than can lead to fractures, pain, and deformity. A link exists between blood pressure and dietary intake of calcium. Some studies show that it can reduce hypertension. It does this most successfully among sodium sensitive individuals: African-

87

Americans, the elderly, and women whose hypertension is pregnancy-induced. Taking calcium supplements and eating a calcium rich diet can minimize that risk, both preventing and treating that disease.

The RDA for calcium is 1000 mg a day for adults, but a higher dosage, 1200 mg, is suggested for postmenopausal women, and pregnant and lactating females. Dairy products, including cheese, yogurt, and milk are good sources of calcium, because they also contain vitamin D and lactose, which aid calcium absorption. Certain greens, such as kale, collards, and broccoli are high in calcium, as are canned fish with edible bones (salmon and sardines). Calcium-fortified bread, cereals, and orange juice are also available.

Even if you eat a lot of calcium-rich food you may deplete your calcium level if the following conditions exist; you are on a high protein or crash diet; or if you fast; drink more than two alcoholic drinks a day; drink four or more cups of coffee a day; smoke; or don't get enough vitamin D. Calcium supplements come in several different forms. Calcium carbonate has the most calcium per tablet and is the cheapest but may not be absorbed well. For those who take medications that decrease stomach acid, calcium citrate may be a better choice. Calcium is best absorbed if supplements are taken in 250 mg to 500 mg doses throughout the day.

Carnitine: Key to Heart Health

Carnitine will help almost every type of cardiovascular disorder: Congestive heart failure, arrhythmias, heart attack, and peripheral vascular disease.

Patients suffering from almost any type of cardiovascular disorder will experience considerable benefit from taking the nutrient **carnitine.** Sometimes known as vitamin B-4, although it is officially not a vitamin, carnitine is essential in the breakdown of fats into energy. There are a variety of carnitines, but only L-carnitine should be taken. Carnitine helps the heart to get sufficient oxygen and to utilize it properly. This amazing substance can bring about improvements in heart health as great as those achieved with drugs. Here's how:

- Carnitine improves the lipid profile by decreasing total cholesterol, lowering triglycerides, and raising the beneficial HDL level. In four months of therapy with L-carnitine, patients experienced on average a 20 percent reduction in total cholesterol, a 28 percent reduction in triglycerides, and a 12 percent increase in HDLs.

- Carnitine helps patients recover more quickly from heart attacks. In research from Italy, a group of heart attack patients were given carnitine and compared with a group who received a placebo. The carnitine patients had improvements in their heart rates and blood pressure, a decrease of angina attacks and rhythm disorders, improvement in the lipid pattern, and a lower mortality rate. Researchers concluded that L–carnitine improves the heart attack patient's condition, quality of life, and life expectancy. Carnitine will also improve heart function in individuals suffering from congestive heart failure. These patients were able to increase their exercise time by 26 percent after receiving carnitine for 180 days, according to one researcher.

- Carnitine acts as a vasodilator, thus helping those who suffer angina attacks by enabling the heart muscle to use oxygen more efficiently. Patients with arrhythmias who take carnitine are often able to reduce their dosages of antiarrhythmic drugs. And carnitine may benefit those with peripheral vascular disease, diabetes, early stage Alzheimer's, Down's syndrome, kidney disease, liver disease, muscular dystrophy, and pulmonary disease. It is thought to be useful for athletes in that it may prolong endurance exercise and lessen muscle fatigue. The usual daily dosage is between 1,500 and 4,000 mg in divided doses. No side effects have been documented from its use.

Carotenoids Explored
Researchers continue to learn more about the health benefits we obtain from the nutrients in fruit and vegetables.

Carotenoids are important nutrients found in vegetables, especially dark green, yellow-orange, and red vegetables, such as tomatoes, spinach, kale, carrots, and sweet potatoes. More than 60 years ago, scientists discovered that a diet rich in carotenoids was inversely related to the number of school days children missed. Researchers learned over the next several decades that consuming fruits and vegetables rich in carotenoids markedly decreased many diseases, particularly cancer. Men with the highest blood levels of carotenoids were one-third less likely to suffer a heart attack than men with the lowest levels.

The most abundant carotenoid is beta-carotene, and for years researchers believed that it was responsible for these benefits. Beta-carotene was hailed for its antioxidant properties and supplementing with it became widespread. Then several major studies appeared indicating that beta carotene supplements offer almost no benefits in protecting against heart disease and cancer; in fact, one study indicated that beta-carotene might play a role in increasing lung cancer among smokers. Researchers looked at their data again and realized that although beta-carotene appeared to be the substances in fruit and vegetables that did the trick, these foods contained many other carotenoids as well as other nutrients. They concluded that it might be one of these other substances, or some combination and interaction among all of them, that creates the positive health effects.

Scientists began studying the role of other carotenoids, such as lycopene, contained in tomatoes, as well as in watermelon and red grapefruit. They found that lycopene was associated with a reduced risk of various deadly cancers such as prostate, colon, and bladder cancer, as well as heart disease. In a 1996 study of male health care professionals, men who ate 10 or more servings of tomatoes weekly were 45 percent less likely to develop prostate cancer. Lutein and zeaxantin, two carotenoids that we get from green leafy vegetables such as spinach and kale, were investigated and found to offer protection against age-related macular degeneration, a deterioration of the retina that can cause blindness. Scientists are still working to determine the effects of the various carotenoids. Although carotenoid supplements exist, the best way to assure an adequate intake is by eating five or more servings of red, dark green, or yellow-orange vegetables daily.

Choline Lowers Cholesterol and More
Choline has also been used successfully to treat head trauma and to improve cognitive and memory disturbances.

Only recently has choline come to be considered an essential nutrient. Choline is necessary for the proper metabolism of fats and the manufacture of a certain neurotransmitter. People fed a choline-deficient diet develop liver problems. In the form of phosphatidylcholine, it increases the solubility of cholesterol, making it less likely to accumulate and cause the blockages that lead to heart attack and stroke. It also inhibits platelet aggregation. In clinical trials in Germany, treatment with phosphatidylcholine lowered cholesterol levels by as much as 28 percent, and triglyceride levels an average of 25 percent. It increased HDL levels 13 to 20 percent. Phosphatidylcholine has been used with success in Europe for treating liver disorders, such as hepatitis, cirrhosis of the liver, and drug-induced liver damage.

But it is best known for aiding brain function. As people age, the choline in the blood does not get into the brain as effectively. Choline increases cerebral metabolism and acts on the levels of various neurotransmitters. It results in improved learning and memory performance in animal models of brain aging. An enthusiastic researcher wrote of it in the publication, *Method and Findings in Experimental Clinical Pharmacology*, saying that it "may be suitable for the treatment of cerebral vascular disease, head trauma of varying severity, and cognitive disorders. In research studies of patients with head trauma, CDP-choline accelerated the recovery from posttraumatic coma and the recuperation of walking ability. It accelerated a better final function result, and reduced the hospital stay of these patients. And it is also credited with improving the cognitive and memory disturbances which are observed after a head trauma of lesser severity and which constitute the disorder known as post concussion syndrome"[41]

Phosphatidylcholine supplementation is reputed to help bipolar depression. It may worsen unipolar depression, however, so patients using it for a depressive disorder should take it only under the supervision of a physician. In one small study in which six patients taking lithium were given the substance, five had substantial reduction in manic symptoms and four had a marked reduction in all mood symptoms during the therapy. Choline exists as a soluble salt or as phosphatidylcholine in lecithin. For lowering cholesterol, 500 to 900 milligrams three times daily of a lecithin product with 90 percent phosphatidylcholine may be prescribed. It is considered safe, although at high doses it may cause gastrointestinal upset. Foods that contain choline include vegetables, egg yolks, beef liver, grains, and legumes.

DHEA: Fountain of Youth?

When taken as a supplement, this hormone may improve memory, enhance sexual functioning, improve immunity and energy, and strengthen the heart.

DHEA (dehydroepiandrosterone) is a hormone produced by the adrenal or stress glands in the body. By age 60, individuals' DHEA levels are

---

[41] Secades, J.J., and Frontera, G., "CDP-choline: Pharmaceutical and clinical review," *Methods and Findings in Experimental Clinical Pharmacology*, vol. 17 (1995).

two-thirds of what they were in their 20s. In addition to decreasing with age, DHEA levels can further decline due to stress, poor diet, lack of exercise, and environmental toxins. One of the ways that DHEA works is by stimulating the activity of cells that fight infection. It boosts immunity to everything from colds to cancer, say its advocates. Low levels of DHEA have been associated with lupus, rheumatoid arthritis, depression, heart disease, high blood pressure, diabetes, and osteoporosis.

DHEA has achieved stardom because it offers so many antiaging benefits. In fact, some researchers think that DHEA will eventually prove to be the fountain of youth. In the last ten years, scientists studying DHEA have come to believe that all the degenerative disorders we experience as we age may be due to the lack of DHEA. By restoring levels to their peak, they say, people can add thirty healthy years to their lives. Studies of mice seem to confirm this theory. Aging mice treated with DHEA were transformed. Their coats became sleek and glossy. Obese mice lost weight. Their immune response improved, their memory was restored, and skin and other cancers were cured. The mice lived longer—in fact their life spans increased by 20 percent. Hundreds of studies have encouraged researchers to believe that similar results can be achieved with humans.

For instance, taken as a supplement, DHEA will improve memory and alertness. It also is reported to increase energy and endurance, reduce stress, and fight depression. When combined with another natural hormone called pregnenolone, DHEA helps form and increase other hormones, especially sex hormones, testosterone in men and estrogen in women. This combination has a strong antiaging effect and is widely reported to increase sexual desire and performance.

An increase in blood levels of DHEA has been associated with a 48 percent reduction in heart disease. This hormone regulates insulin levels and reduces triglyceride levels—two conditions that are risk factors for heart disease and diabetes. DHEA also assists with weight control. It is thought to help the body produce lean muscle tissue rather than fat.

Folic Acid: Nutrient of the '90s
This B vitamin offers strong protection against heart disease, stroke, birth defects, many types of cancers, osteoporosis, and depression.

Until recently, folic acid, a B vitamin also known as folate or folacin, was a relatively ignored nutrient. It has gained fame as the "nutrient of the nineties," however, based on studies that indicate it offers strong protection against an array of disorders. Some experts believe that even a mild deficiency of folic acid may cause 20 to 40 percent of heart attacks and strokes. A modest deficiency in pregnant women can result in certain kinds of birth defects, including the devastating conditions of spina bifida and anencephaly. Low levels of folic acid have been implicated in some types of cancer (including cancer of the colon, cervix, lung, esophagus, and breast) and have also been linked to depression and osteoporosis.

Folic acid prevents heart disease by reducing a person's homocysteine level. When intake of folic acid is low, homocysteine, an amino acid, begins to build up in the blood. At high levels, it is a major risk factor for heart disease, as dangerous as smoking. In the noted Physician's Health Study, researchers discovered that men with the highest homocysteine levels had 3.4 times more heart attacks than those with the lowest levels.[42]

Many other investigations have elucidated the role of homocysteine in cardiovascular disease. An elevated homocysteine level significantly increases the mortality rate among patients undergoing bypass surgery or angioplasty. Blockages in the carotid arteries are a major cause of stroke, and those with high homocysteine levels are more likely than those with low levels, to have these blockages . Supplementation with 400 micrograms of folic acid will readily lower the homocysteine level. Folic acid supplementation will also reduce neural tube defects by 60 to 70 percent. For pregnant women, the recommended dosage is 800 micrograms, and for lactating women, 500 micrograms. So important is this nutrient that the FDA will soon require that flour, breads, and other grain products be fortified with it. A bit of a controversy exists as to whether the planned level of fortification is high enough.

Those using folic acid supplements should also take B-12 supplements because the nutrient can mask an underlying B-12 deficiency. Foods richest in folic acid include fortified cereals (*Total, Grapenuts, All-Bran*), lentils, spinach, chicken livers, peanuts, black and white beans, orange juice, and asparagus.

Ginseng Promotes Vitality

One of the most popular herbs in this country, as well as in the Far East, ginseng has been taken for thousands of years as a sexual restorative for men.

---

[42] Physicians Health Study, a study ongoing since 1982, of data collected from over 20,000 physician-subjects and directed by renowned epidemiologist Dr. Charles Hennekens, professor of Medicine at Harvard Medical School.

Used in the U.S. primarily as a "tonic," ginseng is thought to promote vitality, build stamina, and increase resistance to stress and aging. When college volunteers took 100 mg of ginseng twice daily for 12 weeks, they experienced an improvement in the speed at which they were able to perform mathematical calculations. They did not, however, improve other cognitive or motor functions. Much of the evidence regarding ginseng's qualities is conflicting.

Ginseng contains compounds called ginsenosides, and in test-tube and animal studies these have often produced contradictory effects. Ginsenosides may sometimes raise the blood pressure and sometimes lower it. Sometimes they act as a stimulant and other times as a sedative. Advocates say that this is what makes ginseng a good tonic: it helps the body achieve balance. It does its work by helping the body to adapt, for instance, by regulating temperature or blood pressure up or down, as needed. There is some evidence that ginseng has a beneficial effect on immune function, in both normal patients and patients with depressed cellular immunity, because of either chronic fatigue syndrome or AIDS. Ginseng, along with echinacea, may significantly increase the natural killer cell activity for people in these groups.

Another reason for ginseng's popularity is that it is thought to promote sexual performance and to act as an aphrodisiac. This is indeed true, for studies show that among rodents ginseng "significantly facilitates male copulatory behavior." In humans, however, we have evidence only that it may increase testosterone levels and improve sperm count and motility. Used in the U.S. primarily as a tonic, ginseng may aid the immune system, increase testosterone levels, and may even assist in decreasing the risk of cancer. Ginseng is associated with a decreased risk for cancer. An investigation from Korea indicated that those who consumed ginseng were less likely to get cancer than individuals who did not consume it. A dosage response relationship was also indicated, as the greater the frequency and amount of ginseng intake, the greater the risk reduction. In an animal study ginseng has been demonstrated to reduce the number of tumors and to inhibit their growth.

There are three kinds of ginseng: panax ginseng, the Asian variety; American ginseng, known as panax quinquefolium, and the so-called Siberian ginseng. Asian ginseng may have a stimulant effect that causes insomnia and restlessness as well as high blood pressure. Those individuals with hypertension probably should not take it. American ginseng does not have these side effects, but it is reputed not to have the sexual enhancing properties of the Asian. Both Asian and American ginseng contain ginsenosides. Siberian ginseng, however, is not in the true ginseng genus and does not contain ginsenosides. It is said to be widely used by Russian cosmonauts and athletes to help them improve their stamina and resist stress. The Siberian variety is cheaper than the other types.

Ginseng is expensive: commercial preparations of ginseng cost up to $20 an ounce and vary greatly in quality. Buy a standardized capsule or liquid preparation that specifies the amount of ginsenosides on the label, and buy from a reputable source. In an analysis some years ago of 54 ginseng preparations, 85 percent of them were characterized as worthless for they contained little or no ginseng. Making tea from dried ginseng root is not recommended. Few adverse reactions have been reported from ginseng. It should not be taken with other stimulants or by patients with cardiovascular disease, since reported side effects had included tachycardia and hypertension.

Iron: The Most Common Deficiency

Millions of people, especially women and children, suffer from iron insufficiency with serious health consequences.

Iron deficiency is thought to be the most common nutrient deficiency in the U.S., with an estimated 8 million people suffering from it. Most groups who are at risk are infants, teenage girls, pregnant women (there is a dramatic increase in the need for iron during pregnancy), menstruating women, ethnic minorities, and the elderly. Athletes and vegetarians are also at risk.

You may have a deficiency because you are not eating iron rich foods, or because your body's not absorbing it properly. Bleeding, from excessive menstruation, peptic ulcer, or hemorrhoids, may also cause a deficiency. Weight loss can result in low levels of iron. Healthy obese women who lost weight over a 15-week period saw their iron levels drop significantly, even though they had doubled their intake.

Iron deficiency results in fatigue, irritability, and low resistance to infections. It can lead to anemia, which means the blood is deficient in red blood cells or the hemoglobin portion of red blood cells. Anemia causes extreme fatigue, reduces the body's ability to regulate temperature, weakens the immune system, and lessens the ability to perform physically and mentally. In children, an iron deficiency causes developmental delays and behavior disturbances. In pregnant women, it increases the risk of preterm delivery and a low birth-weight baby.

It is not a good idea to take iron supplements unless you have been found to have a deficiency through a test given by your doctor. There are certain risks involved in having too much iron as well as in having too little. What has made iron supplements controversial in the last few years is that some studies have shown that high levels of iron may play a role in heart disease. Some investigators have suggested that high iron levels increase free radical formation and oxidative stress, which result in athrosclerosis and other damage to the body. In fact, donating blood, which gets rid of some of the body's iron, may help prevent heart attacks—blood donors have an 86 percent lower risk of heart attack than non-donors. Studies are inconsistent and this issue is not yet resolved.

Red meat, especially organ meat, is the major source of iron, but nonetheless it is a good idea to keep it to a minimum in your diet because of other health concerns. There are many other good food sources of iron, including clams, oysters, green leafy vegetables, and whole grains. Most important, choose iron-fortified cereals. Foods rich in vitamin C increase the body's ability to absorb iron, so eat citrus fruits or broccoli at the same time you eat iron rich foods.

Magnesium's Benefits Abound

Some experts have even suggested that magnesium be added to the drinking water in order to reduce the rate of heart disease in the U.S.

There are few nutrients that offer so many diverse benefits to the heart as magnesium. It is estimated that 75 percent of Americans do not receive the Recommended Dietary Allowance of this mineral—and the deficiency is particularly pronounced among the elderly. Magnesium helps the entire cardiovascular system to function properly. It controls the buildup of plaque in the arteries and acts as a vasodilator and an anticoagulant.

A high magnesium level is associated with low blood pressure. Patients should be aware that some hypertensive medications cause further magnesium depletion, and so they should be especially careful to get a sufficient amount of the mineral. Many types of arrhythmias, including atrial fibrillation and ventricular tachycardia, are improved by taking magnesium. Intermittent claudication, the painful leg cramps caused by peripheral vascular disease, is characterized by magnesium deficiency and correcting it can relieve the pain. Magnesium supplements will improve the lipid profile. A deficiency results in lower HDLs and elevated LDLs and triglycerides.

Magnesium is important in the treatment of diabetes, glucose intolerance, insulin resistance, and hypoglycemia, because it assists the body in maintaining proper blood sugar levels. In fact, the American Diabetes Association advises that all persons with diabetes who are at risk for high blood pressure should be treated with magnesium supplements. Magnesium can be an alternative to thrombolytic or "clot busting" therapy after a heart attack. Administration of it intravenously early in the course of a heart attack can reduce the damage. It appears particularly effective in those over age 70.

Magnesium may be useful in treating fibromyalgia, fatigue, glaucoma, hearing loss, osteoporosis, migraine headaches, and kidney stones. Food processing removes magnesium from our diet. And some of the best sources of magnesium are foods we seldom eat: kelp, wheat germ, blackstrap molasses, and brewers yeast. Of the more commonly consumed foods, nuts, especially almonds and cashews, are a good source, as are whole grains and legumes. The recommended dosage in supplement form is 1000 mg, taken separately from calcium.

Omega-3 Essential Fatty Acids Lower Heart Disease Rate

These essential fatty acids prevent the formation of blood clots and plaque, decrease the fibrinogen levels, help arrthymias, and reduce heart attacks.

We need certain fats, called essential fatty acids, to maintain good health and avoid disease. It is estimated that about 90 percent of Americans have a deficiency of essential fatty acids, which may result in many conditions, including fatigue, dry skin and hair, constipation, frequent colds, depression, forgetfulness, and cardiovascular disease.

Omega-3 fatty acids are one type of essential fatty acids and are most important in preventing heart disease. Fish is particularly rich in omega-3s, and most research into this nutrient has been done using fish or fish oils. People who have the highest intake of omega-3 fatty acids, usually through high fish consumption, have the lowest rates of heart attack and cardiovascular disease.

Omega-3 fatty acids lower triglyceride levels and raise the beneficial HDL levels. In addition to these positive effects on the lipid profile, omega-3 fatty acids reduce what is known as "platelet stickiness." When blood platelets adhere to each other, they form the plaque that causes blocked arteries and the clots that break off and travel to the heart causing a heart attack, or to the brain, causing a stroke. The major benefit of omega-3 fatty acids is in lessening these blockages and clots. Among the other positive effects of the omega-3 fatty acids:

- Supplementation with fish oil capsules has been shown to reduce the reclogging of arteries after bypass surgery.
- An investigation of the effect of fish oil capsules on arrhythmias revealed that people taking the fish oil supplements had a 48 percent reduction in the number of extra heartbeats.
- Individuals who eat as little as three ounces of salmon a week according to one study, were half as likely to suffer cardiac arrest as those who did not eat fish rich in omega-3 oils.
- A high fibrinogen level is considered a primary risk factor for heart disease. Omega-3 fatty acids lower the fibrinogen level.

The American Heart Association recommends eating fish rather than taking fish oil capsules. The fish richest in omega-3 fatty acids are sardines, mackerel, salmon, herring, bluefish, whitefish, and halibut. Other experts believe in the efficacy of supplementation with fish oil capsules. Still others say that the benefits of fish oil can be gained by using flaxseed oil (one and a half tablespoons a day, used as salad dressing). At the Cardiovascular Wellness Centers, we recommend the consumption of fish and, frequently, use of an essential oil supplement.

Pantethine Lowers Cholesterol
Pantothenic acid, also known as vitamin B-5, may help rheumatoid arthritis, enhance stamina, and speed recovery after surgery.

When 300 mg were given three times daily to patients with high cholesterol, researchers reported a reduction of total cholesterol by 19 percent, LDL cholesterol by 21 percent, and triglycerides by 32 percent. Furthermore, pantethine increased the beneficial HDL levels by 23 percent. Pantothenic acid, also known as vitamin B-5, is essential for human growth and reproduction. It helps convert fats, carbohydrates, and proteins into energy and aids in the manufacture of adrenal hormones and red blood cells. It is necessary for the normal function of the gastrointestinal tract. All the cells in our body require pantothenic acid.

A derivative of pantothenic acid called pantethine is very beneficial for lowering cholesterol and triglycerides. When 300 mg were given three times daily to patients with high cholesterol, researchers reported a reduction of total cholesterol by 19 percent, LDL cholesterol by

21 percent, and triglycerides by 32 percent. Furthermore, pantethine increased the beneficial HDL cholesterol levels by 23 percent. Even greater are its lipid-lowering effects in diabetics, which it accomplishes without interfering with blood sugar control. The usual dosage of pantethine for cholesterol lowering is 300 mg three times a day. Pantethine works synergistically with two other cholesterol-lowering nutrients, carnitine and CoQ10. These are all contained in the Wellness Centers formulas for cardiovascular health.

Those people with rheumatoid arthritis have lower levels of pantothenic acid than those who do not have the disease, and researchers have found that the lower the level of pantothenic acid the more severe the disease's symptoms. Raising the level of the nutrient may alleviate some of the symptoms of rheumatoid arthritis, and nutritional doctors may prescribe two grams daily for this purpose.

Other uses of pantothenic acid include prescribing it as an "anti-stress vitamin" particularly for those who must undergo severe stress over a long period of time. Some nutritional doctors also use it to treat anxiety and depression. It is sometimes given to athletes and laborers, because it is thought to enhance stamina. There are anecdotal reports of its efficacy in treating certain allergies, and patients who have recently undergone surgery may take it to help rebuild their strength and health.

Good sources of pantothenic acid include brewers yeast, calves liver and other organ meats, as well as fish and poultry, peanuts, mushrooms, soybean flour, split peas, lentils, and broccoli. There is no established recommended daily allowance (RDA) for pantothenic acid, and there are no known side effects or adverse reactions from either pantothenic acid or pantethine. Symptoms of a deficiency of pantothenic acid include fatigue, numbness and shooting pains in the feet, tingling in the hands, headache, and nausea.

Phosphatidylserine Aids Memory
This phospholipid may help you remember where you left your car keys and may improve your ability to concentrate.

Our focus in this section of the book has been on vitamins and other nutrients that are effective in fighting heart disease. There are also nutrients that are known to help to prevent the deterioration that often accompanies aging. In our forties and fifties we may begin to notice that we no longer have the memory we used to have or that our vision gets weaker or sexual performance declines or aches and pains in the joints begin to appear. With each passing decade, these problems may get worse.

Fortunately, we know of natural therapies that can halt or reverse much of this age-related decline. For instance, we too often accept deterioration in mental function as the norm as we get older. But it has been established that people with impaired mental functions and depression often have low levels of phosphatidylserine. This substance, found in the cell membranes of the brain, is what we call a phospholipid. It is concentrated in the cell membrane's outer sheath, which is very important since its structure and function determine what goes in and out of the cell.

Phosphatidylserine is also found in the brain's synapses, the connection between nerve cells that are responsible for inter-cell communication and nerve transmission. There are a number of other key roles that phosphatidylserine plays in the brain. Supplementation with this substance increases the neurotransmitters, which are the little molecules the brain cells use for sending messages to one another. These decrease as we age and in part cause the memory problems. According to research studies, phosphatidylserine will improve your ability to learn names and facts and recall them, recall phone numbers and misplaced objects, and improve the ability to concentrate.

Furthermore, in investigations of patients with Alzheimer's disease, those receiving phosphatidylserine for three months all had improvements in memory, and they were able to maintain the improvements for three months after they stopped taking this nutrient. Research at the prestigious National Institute of Mental Health revealed that healthy people who had age-related memory impairment showed improvement of 15 to 20 percent after treatment with phosphatidylserine.

Selenium Fights Cancer & Heart Disease
People with diets low in this trace mineral have a two to three times greater risk of disease that those with diets rich in it.

Individuals with diets low in selenium have a two to three times greater risk of heart disease than those with diets rich in selenium. This trace mineral is important for heart patients because it performs a number of functions: it acts as an antioxidant, preventing free radical and oxidative damage; it improves the lipid profile, increasing the ratio of the good HDL cholesterol to LDL cholesterol; and it inhibits platelet aggregation (clotting). In one clinical study, patients with blockages of three coronary arteries had low blood selenium levels; those free of blockages had high selenium levels.

But as beneficial as selenium is to heart patients, it is as a cancer fighter that selenium appears to do the most remarkable job. Researchers undertook an investigation of the reported link between selenium and skin cancer. They failed to discover a strong association, but in the course of their work they were astonished to find that patients given selenium had radically reduced rates of several other types of cancer. In patients taking 200 micrograms of selenium daily, the risk of prostate cancer plummeted by 64 percent, colon and rectal cancer dropped by 58 percent, and the lung cancer decreased by 45 percent. The overall mortality rate from cancer among patients taking selenium supplements was 50 percent lower than among people not taking them. Clinical trials are now underway to determine if these findings can be duplicated.

Some investigations have demonstrated that selenium can dramatically improve arthritis. Prostaglandins produce the inflammation of arthritis, and selenium helps to control prostaglandins by controlling the free radical damage that causes their production. Low levels of selenium also have been associated with cataracts, eczema, premature aging, arthritis, and psoriasis. Depressed immune function and impaired resistance to infection have also been attributed to low levels of selenium. Although chronic low levels of this trace mineral are common, a true deficiency is rare and usually occurs in parts of the world where the levels in the soil are low. this results in the risk of a severe heart disorder called Keshan disease.

The amount of selenium in the soil affects the amount of it in the food we eat. The effective forms of the supplement are organic, and include selenium-rich yeast and seleno-methionine. The National Academy of Sciences has established a safe and effective range for selenium of 50 to 200 micrograms daily.

St. John's Wort
St. John's Wort has been used for thousands of years by herbalists to treat a variety of conditions, such as inflammations and viruses.

The herb St. John's Wort received its name because it blooms most profusely on the feast day of St. John, June 24; the word "wort" means plant. The popularity of St. John's Wort has surged recently. Sales of the supplement are 20 times greater than they were just three years ago, and the main reason for this is a 1996 *British Medical Journal* analysis of research that revealed the efficacy of St. John's Wort in relieving depression.[43] In reviewing 23 well-designed clinical trials, investigators concluded that extracts of St. John's Wort are considerably more effective than placebo (dummy pills) for the treatment of mild to moderate depressive disorders. In fact, depressed people taking St. John's Wort were nearly three times as likely to show improvement as those taking a placebo.

When studies compared St. John's Wort to prescription antidepressant medication the results were a tie, with the herb working just as well. (The investigations compared the herb to older types of antidepressants, not the newer selective serotonin reuptake inhibitors such as Prozac and Zoloft. That research remains to be done.) If you suffer from mild to moderate depression, there are good reasons to consider using St. John's Wort. Prescription antidepressants may produce negative side effects, such as sexual dysfunction, fatigue, and diarrhea. The side effects with St. John's Wort are negligible. And St. John's Wort is cheaper: a prescription drug such as Prozac costs about $80 month compared to $10 for St. John's Wort. (Of course, insurance will cover the drug, but not the herb.) Before taking St. John's Wort, however, keep these caveats in mind:

- Its long-term use has not been evaluated. The longest any of these trials lasted was two months.
- The most effective dosage has not been determined.
- Participants in most of the studies suffered mild to moderate depression. Its effect on severe depression is not known.

Vitamin D Deficiency Widespread
Vitamin D is essential for older Americans in order to prevent the bone loss that comes with age and results in crippling fractures.

A study published in the prestigious *New England Journal of Medicine,* reveals that about 40 percent of otherwise healthy Americans residing in the Northeast may not receive enough of the "sunshine vitamin," and among the hospitalized patients, nearly 60 percent were deficient.[44]

---

[43] Linde, K., et al. St. John's Wort for depression—an overview and meta-analysis of randomized clinical trials, *British Medical Journal*, August 3, 1996.
[44] Thomas, M.K., et al., Hypovitaminosis D in medical inpatients, *New England Journal of Medicine*, March 19, 1998.

This discovery has alarmed experts, causing them to reevaluate whether the established recommended daily amount of vitamin D is too low—they've found that even those people taking supplements with vitamin D have insufficient quantities of it in their bodies.

Why is vitamin D important? It is needed because it helps our bones absorb calcium and slows bone loss. In its most severe form, a deficiency of vitamin D can cause rickets in children. But the lack of this vitamin can have disastrous consequences for older people, causing bone loss, osteoporosis, and the devastating fractures that cripple so many. Vitamin D may also be important to muscle function, immune defenses, and even in preventing certain kinds of cancers. Exposure to sunlight helps the body to make vitamin D. People who live in a tropical climate probably have enough of it. But those residing in less sunny climes (the research was done in Boston) are likely to have a deficiency, particularly in the winter if they stay indoors, or if they go outside and cover most of their skin. As people get older they require more vitamin D. Among a group of hospitalized patients in the study, 57 percent were vitamin D deficient, 22 percent severely. Nearly half of those who said they took vitamin D regularly were nonetheless deficient. The problem is not only in hospitalized people. In another study of healthy people under 65 years of age, 42 percent lacked a sufficient amount of vitamin D.

The Nutrition Board of the Institutes of Medicine has recommended an intake of 200 IU [international units] daily for people 19 to 50, 400 IU daily for those 51 to 70, and 600 IU daily for those 71 and older. But experts are now suggesting that adults probably need 800 to 1000 IUs daily. It's difficult to get this amount from food, and vitamin D is usually not sold as a stand-alone vitamin. Experts recommend that it be made available as a stand-alone vitamin and that the amount in multivitamins, calcium supplements, and fortified foods be increased. Foods that contain vitamin D include oily fish, such as tuna, salmon, as well as eggs. Milk and many kinds of cereals are fortified with vitamin D.

Chapter Seven
Questions & Answers

Human Growth Hormone (HGH) and the Advance of Preventive Medicine

Human Growth Hormone is one of many endocrine hormones like estrogen, progesterone, testosterone, melatonin, and DHEA (dehydroepiandrosterone), which the body produces for specific purposes in directing metabolism. It is composed of a combined series of amino acids and emanates from the pituitary gland to promote cell growth. It is the most abundant hormone produced by the pituitary gland, but its secretions diminish with age. At age 60, HGH secretions are about 25 percent of what they were at 20. Discovered as early as 1912, it has been approved for use in treating pituitary gland disorders that retard growth; e.g., dwarfism. Research in the last 20 years has shown that HGH hormone replacement offers many benefits that counter the aging process, and it has become a leading therapy in antiaging medicine.

A list of the demonstrated physical benefits of HGH replacement therapy includes restoring muscle mass, decreasing body fat, thickening the skin and reducing wrinkles, restoring lost hair, restoring hair color, increasing energy, increasing sexual function, improving cholesterol profile, restoring size of liver, pancreas, heart, and other organs that shrink with age, improving vision, improving memory, elevating mood and improving sleep, normalizing blood pressure, increasing cardiac output and stamina, improving immune function, and assisting in wound healing.

The following are questions regarding the subject of Human Growth Hormone excerpted from an interview I gave on my radio program.

Q: *Human growth hormone (HGH) has been under study by the FDA for more than three years, and it has been popularized in a number of books and research papers for two decades. Do you think that* *awareness of the product will grow among the public and that it will become a mainstream therapy?*

A: What the drive behind HGH research today stems from is the product market. There are a number of human growth hormone *boosters* or *precursors* being promoted in the mainstream media—radio, TV, print advertisements. It is also being promoted in the bodybuilding community. This kind of health information will gradually increase awareness of HGH among the general public. Even though the research has been going on for more than 20 years, relatively few people know about HGH and its many benefits.

Books like *Grow Young with HGH* by Dr. Ronald Klatz,[45] a colleague of mine, which came out in 1998, have made growth hormone very well known among persons familiar with the American Academy of Anti-Aging Medicine.[46] As early as 1990, Dr. Daniel Rudman published the results of his research in the *New England Journal of Medicine*. He describes how replacing the human growth hormone—which gradually recedes with age—results in an array of youthful benefits in the body: skin is thickened, lean body mass replaces fatty stores, energy gets a boost, and all organ functions show improvement. There are other studies in the literature that focus on how the growth hormone may correct certain organ failure conditions, such as cardiomyopathy and heart failure.

Q: *Many people have taken melatonin and DHEA when these became popular therapies. Will these people move up to HGH therapy, or are certain therapies more appropriate for one person than another? In other words, will HGH therapy replace the other two?*

A: Melatonin is a hormone of the pineal gland—the gland set in the cranium behind and between your eyes. It has been touted as a powerful antioxidant with all attendant benefits as a cancer fighter, heart helper, and energy enhancer. It became popular as a sleep aid and an antidote to jet lag. Because the pineal gland is the "timekeeper of the brain," it keeps track of our body's daily and seasonal rhythms. Growth hormone would be a complement to melatonin. There is a synergistic effect when the body's hormones work together. DHEA is quite different. It is a product of the adrenal gland. It is the most abundant hormone in the human body and

---

[45] Katz, Dr. Ronald, *Grow Young with HGH*, HarperCollins Publishers, 1997.
[46] D. Rudman, D., et al., "Effects of Human Growth Hormone," *New England Journal of Medicine*, July 5, 1990.

is involved in the manufacture of the sex hormones, estrogen, and testosterone. It also promotes the release of the growth hormone in the way that all hormones work together. A comprehensive antiaging therapy program would include all of these modalities, plus testosterone for men and estrogen and progesterone for women.

Q: *Then it would not be redundant for women already taking hormones or for men already on testosterone to take growth hormone therapy. Is that correct?*

A: Let's make a couple of clarifications and distinctions at this juncture. All of the researchers in the field of antiaging and human growth hormone are also users of growth hormone therapy. Dr. Alan Ahlschier comes to mind. He is a board-certified family practice physician and radiologist, who is also a consultant in antiaging medicine. He tells of dozens of personal health improvements as a result of growth hormone therapy, including better muscle tone, improved vision, and a better mental outlook. "I never get sick. I feel so much younger than I ever did before," he told me. I can attest to the same feelings from my own growth hormone therapy. It involves taking a product I was instrumental in designing and have endorsed for the manufacturer: *Chronogenics.*

Chronogenics is in a class of product called *secretagogues* or growth hormone *boosters* or *precursors.* Human growth hormone is not easily obtained. For its earliest approved use as a cure for hypopituitary dwarfism (children who do not grow normally), it had to be extracted from cadavers. In the 1980s Genentech and Eli Lilly Pharmaceuticals succeeded in producing it in the lab by DNA technology; that is, splicing and recombining genetic elements. But "recombinant HGH," is expensive and difficult to administer and control. Secretagogues are combinations of various amino acids, which prompt the pituitary gland to secrete natural growth hormone and promote its effectiveness. Chronogenics, which I take as a tablet, is one of these and it is also considerably less expensive than injections of recombinant HGH. Injections of recombinant growth hormone could cost thousands of dollars. Many hormone replacements are not covered by insurance. Estrogen is covered. Testosterone could be covered where indicated. Melatonin and DHEA are not nor are the boosters, but their introduction has made growth hormone therapy available at moderate cost.

Q: *With respect to heart disease, it is not clear from the literature whether it is beneficial or a risk. How do you deal with a heart disease patient who wishes to take HGH therapy hormones? Is there careful monitoring involved?*

A: With regards to aging and heart disease, it has never been shown scientifically that low HGH levels are associated with heart disease. But today we know much more about the etiology of heart disease. For example, we're studying endothelial dysfunction, an unhealthy condition of the inner lining of the arteries that allows plaque to build up. It could be inferred that anything that promotes overall bodily health, as growth hormone does, will make the heart and arteries function better. In a well know European study involving 333 patients with severe growth hormone deficiency, researchers found that they had twice the mortality rate compared to a group matched for age and sex. They found that the group of 333 tended to be overweight, have a poor fat-to-lean body ratio, and also to have elevated cholesterol levels. Each of these risk factors would be reduced with growth hormone therapy.

There have also been studies where patients with cardiomyopathy, or a weak heart were given HGH and their condition improved. In 1996, an article in the *New England Journal of Medicine*[47] reported the results of a study in which researchers administered growth hormone to seven patients with moderate to severe heart failure. The growth hormone increased the thickness of the left ventricular wall of patients, which makes the heart function better, pump blood easier, and increases exercise capacity. When you consider that there is no truly successful treatment for reversing heart failure, this occurrence was remarkable and promising. There has also been much study of testosterone and heart disease, showing that the hormone helps the coronary arteries dilate and increases overall stamina.

Q: *There are dozens of new products promoted in advertisements these days with claims to provide benefits to specific problems, e.g., hair growth, improved eyesight, wrinkle removal, better memory, greater sexual function, weight loss, etc. Are these new products offshoots of hormone research and HGH science?*

---

[47] Turner, H., et al., "Growth Hormone in the Treatment of Dilated Cardiopyopathy," *New England Journal of Medicine,* August 29, 1996.

A: That's all in the power of advertising. Some of it is a false claim. But some of them are of value; there's a CoQ10 cream, and an antioxidant cream, for example. It's a multi-billion dollar business. It's logical that many products would derive from the antiaging research. The antiaging movement has made people think about restoring youthful characteristics—skin, hair, libido, and mental sharpness. In many instances, there is a basis in research being done on natural hormones as well as nutrients for these self-improvement products. Many nutrients help cerebral function: ginkgo biloba, phosphatidylserine, vinco pincitene, and the like. It remains to be seen whether some of them will be successful. Unless there is sound scientific research behind them, they will eventually fail in the marketplace.

Q: *You are a member of the American Academy of Anti-Aging Medicine. What role do you play in the organization? How much of your practice is dedicated to antiaging medicine? Have you become an antiaging educator?*

A: The American Academy of Anti-Aging Medicine[48] is an organization of 10,000 physicians and scientists from sixty countries, founded in 1993 in Chicago and is dedicated to the advancement of therapeutics related to the science of longevity medicine. I've been a member since 1996. I have been designated by the president as one of the premier antiaging physicians in the country. I specialize in cardiovascular antiaging medicine. I have spoken at the international annual meetings and my writings appear in the Academy's publications.

What I do and have been doing in my practice is in fact antiaging, because antiaging medicine is essentially preventive medicine. You stay young by preventing degenerative diseases. You do that through early detection, lifestyle changes, the right diet and exercise—and now as science carries us further along—through the use of hormone replacement medicine, such as HGH and the other hormones we have discussed here. As part of my analysis, I do a hormonal evaluation. But since HGH itself is extremely irregular in its secretions throughout the day, to evaluate it requires measuring a parallel hormone, IGF-1 (Insulin Growth Factor 1). As its name implies, IGF-1 is a hormone resembling insulin. It parallels the growth hormone in its activities except that its levels are more easily

---

[48] See the home page of the American Board of Anti-Aging Medicine, www.worldhealth.net/index/shtml.

measurable. Its desirable level should be around 350 as we age. In many patients however, we see levels as low as 80 or 90, which would be the normal growth hormone levels of a person 90 or 100 years old. Patients often present tired and fatigued beyond what their age actually is. By boosting those levels, we see definite improvement of a patient's overall health.

Q: *Is HGH therapy a long-term commitment, like having to take insulin if you are a diabetic? People are always concerned about side effects. HGH may be natural, but nature shut it down, perhaps for a good reason. Can the risk be reduced to zero or to parity with statins? What successes have there been in measuring the levels of HGH in patients? Isn't this key to controlling HGH therapy for maximum benefits?*

A: HGH therapy could be a long time commitment, like insulin replacement for diabetics. When dosages are carefully controlled there is very little danger of side effects. If there were a dangerous side effect, it would be cancer. Growth hormone promotes cell growth and it would promote cancerous cell growth if cancer were present. There is no evidence, however, that growth hormone induces cancer. The risk is very low. I would say not greater than that of taking cholesterol medications.

We monitor patients through blood tests every three months. People come into this office with or without heart disease. We see people who are tired, depressed, have muscle weakness, and chronic high blood pressure, and men who have declining sexual activity. If they have a heart problem, these symptoms are intensified. We measure their antiaging biomarkers, and then we not only treat the heart, but we offer hormone therapy. Often when we tell them their growth hormone is low, they will say "no thanks I don't want to keep growing." That's when we have to do some health education.

Chapter Eight
Natural Therapies

Reduce Cholesterol

My primary goal in treating elevated cholesterol levels is to successfully lower them with natural therapies. I do, of course, give drug therapy to patients who have severe problems or who are not compliant with a natural cholesterol-lowering regimen. I especially urge younger patients to try natural therapies because I don't like to begin them on a course of drugs that they will have to stay with for thirty or forty years. Older patients who are not symptomatic can also benefit from natural therapies. Even those patients who must take drugs will be able to cut back on the dosage if they use supplements in combination with medication.

In my experience, most dietary management, such as the American Heart Association's Step 1 and Step 2 diets, result in only minimal benefits unless combined with supplements. An insulin-regulating (low carbohydrate) diet is extremely effective for patients with insulin problems and those who have that cluster of symptoms that includes high triglycerides, high blood pressure, central abdominal obesity, and low levels of the beneficial HDL cholesterol. Vegetarian diets can be excellent for reducing cholesterol, but some patients may have to take certain precautions with them, and be careful not to overconsume carbohydrates. Here are the natural therapies I recommend to my patients with elevated cholesterol levels:

- **Niacin** (500-1500 mg): Niacin had long been the first line of defense against high cholesterol, but it has lost some of its popularity in recent years because of its side effects. I find, however, that niacin can be very effective, but it must be used carefully. It is particularly beneficial if the patient has high total cholesterol along with high triglycerides and low HDL cholesterol.

    There are two types of niacin: immediate release and time-release. I use a good amount of time-release niacin, which must be closely monitored, because it can cause liver damage. Niacin also is known to cause flushing, but this can be avoided with the time-release type. Other side effects include stomach problems, arrhythmias, alterations in blood sugar, and rashes. I don't prescribe more that 1500 mg, and I find that if it is used with magnesium and chromium its benefits are further enhanced.

- **Chromium** (200-600 micrograms): This trace mineral is especially effective in reducing insulin resistance, raising the level of beneficial HDL cholesterol, and lowering triglycerides.
- **Magnesium** (500-1000 mg): Magnesium not only causes cholesterol levels to fall, it helps the entire cardiovascular system function better. It will improve blood pressure and help some arrhythmias.
- **Soy**: It's easy to incorporate soy into your diet, or you can take it as a supplement: three soy capsules or two scoops of soy powder in a glass of water daily.
- **Fiber complex**: We need 30 grams of fiber a day and most Americans are not getting that from their diets. Taking a fiber supplement, such as psyllium, oat bran, or guar, will not only help lower cholesterol but will assist in reducing blood pressure and blood insulin levels.
- **Pantethine** (450-900 mg): Pantethine offers a quadruple whammy in improving lipids: it will cause total cholesterol, LDL cholesterol, and triglycerides to drop, while raising the beneficial HDL cholesterol level.
- **Lecithin and choline** (3 capsules, 500-900 mg): This nutrient increases the solubility of cholesterol, which decreases its ability to cause atherosclerosis. In one study, high doses of it lowered total cholesterol by 33 percent and raised HDLs by 46 percent.
- **Garlic**: Garlic's benefits can be obtained by consuming one-half to one clove a day or by taking three to six capsules as a supplement.
- **L-carnitine** (500-1000 mg): This nutrient helps decrease total cholesterol and is especially effective in lowering triglycerides. In addition, it may help angina, arrhythmias, congestive heart failure, diabetes, and assist with recovery after a heart attack.
- **Essential oils-EPA** (fish oil) and **GLA** (evening primrose, black currant, or borage oil), 3 capsules a day: These oils have many heart benefits in addition to cholesterol reduction. They help to lower blood pressure and to prevent the development of dangerous blood clots.
- **High potency antioxidants**: Those such as vitamins C and E are key in stopping the damage caused by LDL cholesterol.

- **Other nutrients**: As part of our cholesterol reduction program are *gugulipids* (an Indian herb), 640-1500 mg; *tocotrienal,* 100-300 mg; and *plant phytosterols* (250-1000 mg). Despite all the therapies available to assist in reducing cholesterol and despite the education efforts made by the medical community and the government, cholesterol levels among the U.S. population remain very high. Only 18 percent of heart patients reach the cholesterol-lowering goals set by their physicians, according to a recent survey. Furthermore, there are indications that those target cholesterol levels may not be low enough—the standard cholesterol guidelines need revising downward. [See New Cholesterol Guidelines in Chapter One.] New research shows that patients whose cholesterol falls within the "normal" range can benefit from additional cholesterol reduction. Cholesterol-lowering is one of the most effective means for combating heart disease, which kills one out of three Americans. As I often tell my patients, don't wait until you are in the ICU with a heart attack to say, "Gee, I should have done that."

A new natural therapy for lowering cholesterol

At the Wellness Centers, we have had great success with a new natural therapy that can replace drugs for many patients with mildly to moderately elevated cholesterol. A supplement containing *red yeast rice* may enable patients with cholesterol levels in the 200 to 240 mg/DL range to stay off cholesterol-lowering prescription medication. This supplement is safe, cheaper than drugs, and has fewer side effects. It should be taken in combination with diet and exercise

Red yeast rice has been used for centuries in China in the making of rice wine, as a food preservative and flavor enhancer, as well as for medicinal purposes. In recent years, scientists discovered that red yeast rice contains HMGCoA reductase inhibitors, which are the key ingredient in the cholesterol-lowering drug Lovastatin. This finding led researchers to study red yeast rice's cholesterol-lowering properties, which were discovered to be significant. Red yeast rice was brought to market as a dietary supplement only within the past three years.

In a clinical trial, 446 patients with total cholesterol levels of about 230 mg/DL were given two capsules of red yeast rice extract for eight weeks. The patients maintained their normal lifestyle and dietary habits, although they received nutritional counseling. After eight weeks, the total cholesterol levels were reduced an average of 23 percent. LDL cholesterol was lowered by 28.5 percent and triglycerides by 36.5 percent. The beneficial HDL cholesterol increased by 19.6 percent. Few adverse effects occurred. Six people said they experienced heartburn, and three said they had a feeling of abdominal flatulence.

A second study, a randomized, double-blind, placebo-controlled trial, used red yeast rice with 152 patients with cholesterol levels of about 250 mg/DL. After eight weeks, those patients who got the red yeast rice had a total cholesterol reduction on average of 19 percent compared to only 1.5 percent among those who did not receive the substance. Triglycerides levels plunged an average of 36 percent for the red yeast rice patients, compared to 9 percent in the placebo group. LDL levels were reduced an average of 27 percent and the beneficial HDL levels increased by over 16 percent.

Although we have excellent medicines to lower cholesterol, many people don't like the idea of being on drug therapy for a lifetime. Unfortunately, there could be a problem with red yeast rice, since the FDA may prevent its import, and it will no longer be available in nutritional supplements. The Wellness Centers use a natural based formula called Cholesterol Control, which, along with a program of diet and exercise, is very beneficial and effective in lowering cholesterol. Another natural substance to consider is Policosanol, which has come into the forefront as a natural cholesterol-lowering agent. It is an extract of sugar cane and appears to have an anti-platelet effect on the blood vessel walls. Policosanol is currently being used in the Wellness Centers' program of cholesterol lowering through natural means.

Lower Blood Pressure

In my practice, I saw a woman in her sixties with high systolic blood pressure (between 170 and 190), who did not want to go on blood pressure medication. She falls into the category of the type of patient that I see more and more often: those who want to try holistic therapy to control hypertension. In my practice, I offer a program that includes diet, exercise, and vitamins, and it very often enables patients to avoid drug therapy.

There are a variety of reasons why patients don't want blood pressure medication. Patients are more informed than they used to be, and they know there are better ways to deal with high blood pressure than to go on a lifetime program of taking drugs. Many patients who are currently on blood pressure pills have a lot of complications, such as constipation, peripheral edema, and sexual dysfunction. They would like to find another way to control their hypertension.

I want to very clearly make the point that I do use many drugs in my practice. With very high blood pressure, or when the patient has other complications, it is essential to get the blood pressure down as quickly as possible. But with the majority of patients, we can first try natural therapies. This will require a commitment on the part of the patient; a program of natural therapies demands more discipline than just swallowing a pill.

What I see most frequently in patients at the Wellness Centers is hypertension with obesity. If these patients lose weight, their blood pressure will often go to normal. If it doesn't go to normal, it will at least go to lower levels, and they'll require less drug therapy. The majority of patients coming in to see me also have the insulin problems that characteristically accompany obesity and hypertension. These patients do well on the Wellness Centers' insulin-regulating diet, which is low in carbohydrates and fat.

The American Heart Association recommends the DASH diet for hypertensive patients.[49] This salt-restricting diet is rich in fruits and vegetables and in fat-free or low-fat dairy products. It was found to produce the greatest reduction in systolic and diastolic blood pressure. I believe the DASH diet is most suitable for those hypertensive patients who do not have insulin disorders. For those with insulin disorders, let me warn you that one of the big offenders I see in these patients are the excessive use of fruits. Fruits contain a lot of sugar, and sugar must be restricted for those with insulin disorders.

Keep in mind that finding the right diet is not a simple matter, and no one diet is right for everyone. Your physician should be working with you on your diet. It should be individualized and monitored. It's not enough for doctors to give patients a piece of paper that says eat turkey and lettuce. Nutritional counseling is very important. In addition to weight reduction and an insulin-regulating diet, we strongly recommend an exercise program. You don't have to go a health club or buy expensive equipment—although you can if you want to. We like to prescribe fast walking

---

[49] *DASH diet,* the eating plan from the "Dietary Approaches to Stop Hypertension" clinical study. The research was funded by the National Heart, Lung, and Blood Institute (NHLBI), with additional support by the National Center for Research Resources and the Office of Research on Minority Health, all units of the National Institutes of Health. DASH's final results appear in the April 17, 1997, issue of the New England Journal of Medicine. The results show that the DASH "combination diet" lowered blood pressure and, so, may help prevent and control high blood pressure. www.nhlbi.nih.gov/health/public/heart/hbp/dash.

or other aerobic exercises at least 20 minutes a day, working up to an hour a day every day. Stress management techniques and relaxation therapies, such as meditation, yoga, or biofeedback are extremely important in lowering blood pressure, and we recommend that our patients find a way to work these disciplines into their daily life.

Needless to say, smoking cessation, which is essential for everyone, is particularly critical for those with high blood pressure. One research effort showed that hypertensive men who smoke have twenty times the risk of stroke as nonsmokers. It's also important to limit alcohol intake if you have high blood pressure. Men should have not more than 10 oz. of wine daily and women, 5 oz.

The following is a list of the supplements we recommend to be taken daily for hypertension, but we do not suggest that you follow this unless you have consulted your own doctor or a clinical nutritionist. When we recommend potassium and magnesium, we must make sure there is no problem with renal insufficiency.

- Magnesium, 500 - 3000 mg
- Taurine, 1000 - 3000 mg
- Arginine, 1000 -3000 mg
- Garlic, 3 - 6 capsules
- Calcium, 1000 mg at night
- Essential oil formulation, 3 or 4 capsules
- Primrose or borage oil, 1000 mg three times per day
- CoQ1O, 50 - 200 mg
- Potassium, 99 milliequivalents, one to three times per day
- Hawthorn, three capsules per day
- Fiber formula
- Chromium, 200 - 1000 micrograms

These are the key elements of the Wellness Centers' program for controlling high blood pressure naturally. Let me repeat: this program does require a commitment on the part of the patients. But those who make the commitment will almost certainly see a payoff in better health.

Alleviate Arrhythmias

When treating arrhythmias, we try the simplest therapy first. Most arrhythmias are not dangerous, but they may cause the patient discomfort or alarm. Nutritional therapy alone may alleviate these benign arrhythmias. In the case of the more serious arrhythmias, we use natural therapies in conjunction with drugs or other treatments; this often enables patients to decrease the amount of medicines they take. Even when they fail to "cure" the arrhythmias, nutritional remedies may lessen their frequency, duration, and intensity. Listed below are the nutrients we prescribe for our patients with rhythm disorders.

- **Magnesium, calcium, and potassium**: Magnesium is essential in treating arrhythmias; in fact, a magnesium deficiency may be the cause of the arrhythmia. Often this deficiency will occur if the patient is taking diuretics, which drain the body of magnesium and other nutrients as well. Magnesium supplements should be taken in conjunction with calcium, since it's important to establish a balance between these two minerals. Magnesium depletion in the heart muscle can also result in potassium depletion. These electrolytes are needed for proper nerve and muscle firings, so potassium must also be kept at adequate levels and in balance. Magnesium is safe for many types of arrhythmias including atrial fibrillation, ventricular tachycardia, and ventricular premature contractions. Try to get magnesium from your diet as well as from supplements by eating dark green leafy vegetables, whole grains, legumes, and nuts. Green leafy vegetables will also provide potassium, as will citrus fruits, bananas, and potatoes.
- **Omega 3 fatty acids**: As described in Chapter Six, omega-3 fatty acids offer amazing benefits to the heart, and among the ways they work is by preventing arrhythmias. One investigation found that people taking fish oil capsules had a 48 percent reduction in the number of extra heartbeats. Another dramatic study indicated that people who eat as little as three ounces each week, of fish such as salmon (rich in Omega 3s), were half as likely to suffer cardiac arrest, a condition caused by the arrhythmia known as ventricular fibrillation. Other heart benefits from fish and fish oil include lower blood pressure, low cholesterol and triglycerides, and fewer dangerous blood clots that lead to heart attack and stroke.
- **Selenium**: This micronutrient as described in Chapter Six, known primarily as a cancer fighter, can also help rhythm disorders. In one investigation, patients with long-term, low levels of selenium who had arrhythmias and other cardiac disorders showed significant improvement (and in one case the arrhythmia disappeared dramatically) after supplementing with selenium. In

animal studies, selenium supplementation induced a significant reduction in the severity of arrhythmias. In addition to taking supplements, you can add selenium to your diet by eating bran, tuna fish, tomatoes, and broccoli.

- **L-carnitine**: An amino acid that we prescribe for controlling hypertension and for lowering cholesterol, L-carnitine may ameliorate arrhythmias as well. In a study of 160 patients who had experienced a heart attack, those who received a daily dose of L-carnitine for a year afterwards had fewer rhythm disorders than those who did not. In another research effort, patients with angina and arrhythmias who took L-carnitine were able to reduce the amount of their antiarrhythmic drugs. They also had improvement in their blood pressure, lipid pattern, and degree of their angina attacks.
- Other nutrients that will assist in eliminating arrhythmias and promote the general health of the cardiovascular system include zinc, co-enzyme Q1O, and taurine.

Some simple lifestyle changes will get rid of many arrhythmias. Cutting back on the intake of sweets, including fruit juices, may help. Eliminating caffeine, cigarettes, and excessive alcohol from the diet is also important. Hospital emergency rooms often see people over the Christmas and New Year's holidays with arrhythmias brought on by excessive alcohol consumption. Stress and acute anger may trigger arrhythmias; so learning to avoid or deal with the emotional disturbances in life is important. Since rhythm disorders are sometimes due to thyroid problems, you may want to ask your doctor for a thyroid test. Many types of medications, including diet pills and cold medicines, can cause arrhythmias. Those who experience rhythm disorders should ask their physician to evaluate their medication.

Control Diabetes, Glucose, and Insulin

The majority of patients with Type 2 diabetes can probably keep their disease under control through a proper nutritional program, exercise, and weight loss. If they are diligent about making lifestyle changes and staying with a program, they can dramatically reduce the complications of their disease. They may never have to take insulin or any type of medication. Although Type 1 diabetics will always have to use insulin, they can greatly decrease the amount they take as well as the dangerous consequences of the disease. Some basics:

- **Diet and weight loss.** While we emphasize the important role supplements can play in controlling diabetes, they cannot work in the absence of a carefully planned and maintained diet. All diabetics should be on an individualized eating plan to normalize their blood sugar levels as well as to help them lose weight. Among the most important dietary adjustments they must make are to eliminate most sugar and simple carbohydrates, eat little saturated fat, and curb the intake of processed foods. Instead, they need plenty of fiber from whole grains; lots of vegetables, especially broccoli and other cruciferous vegetables, and some fruit, but not an excessive amount. Particularly healthy for diabetics are fish and some soy products.
- **Exercise.** Exercise increases insulin sensitivity and offers cardiovascular benefits in terms of decreases in blood pressure, cholesterol, and triglyceride levels. It promotes weight loss and helps with fatigue.
- **Control blood pressure.** Controlling blood pressure will cut the risk of diabetic complication by about 25 percent and reduce the risk of dying from diabetes-related illness by almost a third.
- **No smoking and little alcohol.** Diabetics who smoke have a dramatic increase in risk of heart attack and high risk for kidney damage. They should keep their alcohol intake to a minimum because it worsens their glucose tolerance.
- **Education and therapy.** Depression is common among diabetics, and unfortunately, they achieve poor results with antidepressant drugs or have side effects from them. Psychotherapy may not only alleviate the depression, but also may help patients manage their diabetes. When the psychotherapy is combined with a diabetes education program, it is even more effective. At the Wellness Centers, we offer a program of nutrition, education, and support for diabetes patients. In many communities, hospitals may provide similar programs. Take advantage of such programs if they are available. Managing diabetes is tough, but if you conscientiously utilize the information and tools available, you can live a normal, long, and healthy life.

Vitamins, minerals, and other nutrients can play a major role in controlling diabetes. Taken as supplements, they work in a variety of ways. Some nutrients improve glucose tolerance or help to process glucose. Others increase the diabetic's sensitivity to insulin. Still other nutrients are successful in preventing or reducing nerve damage or pain from nerve damage or they offer antioxidant protection against free radicals—especially important for diabetics.

Furthermore, the nutrients that help diabetes are also beneficial for the vast number of people with glucose intolerance or insulin resistance. If a person has high blood pressure, high triglycerides, and a fat stomach, he or she probably also has insulin resistance and/or glucose intolerance. All of these conditions are part of a syndrome known as Syndrome X, which leads not only to diabetes but also puts people at high risk for heart disease.

Lipoic acid is just one example of a natural substance that is very effective for diabetes and related conditions. It has been found to improve diabetic neuropathy (loss of nerve function characteristic of diabetes), mainly because of its antioxidant properties but also because it improves blood sugar metabolism, helps blood flow to the peripheral nerves, and even stimulates the regrowth of nerve fibers. In one study, patients taking 600 mg of lipoic acid daily reported an 82.5 percent decrease in their symptoms within nineteen days. In fact, diabetics must be careful with lipoic acid because, if they also take drugs or insulin, their dosage requirements may be significantly reduced.

Biotin, a B vitamin, is another nutrient that offers many benefits to these patients. Researchers report that supplementing with biotin can cause significant drops in blood sugar levels—by about 50 percent in some studies. Biotin will also enhance insulin sensitivity and reduce pain from diabetic nerve damage. Like lipoic acid, biotin may require readjusting the patient's medication. Certain herbs, such as fenugreek, which supports healthy glucose metabolism, can also help these patients. These are only a few of about a score of nutrients that offer amazing benefits to diabetics and others with insulin problems. (See supplement listing in this section.)

Supplement Recommendations

These nutrients will not only help control diabetes, they may prevent its development when taken by those with glucose intolerance or insulin resistance – both prediabetic conditions. Amounts to be taken daily:

Vitamin E :	400-1200 LU
Lipoic acid:	50-300 mg
Biotin:	5-100 mg
Chromium:	200-1000 mcg
Vitamin C:	500-3,000 mg
B-6 :	50-100 mg
B-12:	1000-3000 mcg
Essential fatty acids:	3 tablets/day (1000 mg of fish oil 3x daily with meals.)
Fenugreek:	300 mg
Gymnema sylvestre:	100 mg
Magnesium:	500-2000 mg
Zinc:	25-200 mg
Coenzyme Q10:	50-300 mg
Inositol:	500-2000 mg
Carnitine:	500-2000 mg
Selenium:	200 mcg
Manganese:	30 mg
Bioflavonoids:	1,000-2,000 mg
Potassium:	100 multi-equivalents
Pyridoxine:	50-150 mg

Spur Weight Loss

Patients are often surprised to learn that one of the ways we attack their overweight condition is through a program of vitamins, minerals, and other nutrients. These natural therapies must be part of an overall program that includes diet and exercise if they are to be truly effective. We use natural therapies to affect the body's processes in many different ways. Some nutrients are *fat burners* or *fat blockers*. Others suppress the appetite or boost energy. Still others help with weight loss by stabilizing intestinal flora. Hormone therapy also plays a role. Although we have divided these nutrients into different categories depending on how they work in the body, many of them perform several different actions. Here are some of the key nutrients for weight loss.

Fat burners: These help increase the body's metabolic rate so that calories are burned up faster.

Among the most effective fat burners are:
- **L-tyrosine**: This amino acid works by stimulating production of adrenaline, thereby allowing the body to burn fat faster.
- **Ephedrine**: Contained in the herb *ma huang*, ephedrine keeps the metabolic rate elevated and helps the body burn extra calories during exercise. Ephedrine has been a subject of controversy lately because it can cause serious problems if it is taken in large quantities. Persons with heart disease should not take ephedrine, especially if they have an irregular heartbeat. Others may use it cautiously, in consultation with a nutritional physician.
- **Gamma linolenic acid**: Contained in borage oil, flaxseed, and evening primrose, this essential fatty acid helps accelerate fat loss by contributing to the production of thyroid and growth hormones, two important regulators of normal fat metabolism.
- **Sodium pyruvate** or pyruvic acid. A favorite of body builders, pyruvate prevents carbohydrates from turning into fat and keeps the metabolism in high gear.
- **L-carnitine**: The body requires carnitine in order to properly use fat for energy.

Fat blockers. Nutrients in this category hinder absorption of fat in the intestine.
- Most notable for performing this function are **fiber complex** and **chitosan,** a substance derived from oyster shells.

Energy Enhancers. One of the main problems of overweight people is fatigue. They've lost their get-up-and-go and are too tired to participate in physical activity. They develop a sedentary lifestyle, which then further adds to their overweight condition. To combat fatigue, use:
- **Ginseng**: This root has been taken as a tonic for centuries. The best selling herb in the U.S., thousands of users attest to its efficacy in improving energy levels and general well-being. Trials have shown that it also aids athletic performance.
- **Coenzyme Q1O**: This is an essential component of the mitochondria, the energy-producing unit of the cells of our body. Among its many uses are to improve chronic fatigue and to aid athletic performance.

- **Vitamin B-12**: Known as the energy vitamin, B-12 has long been used to combat fatigue and anemia in those who have a deficiency.

Insulin regulators/appetite suppressants. If a person is insulin resistant, as a majority of overweight people are, these nutrients will increase insulin sensitivity, which improves not only blood sugar control but also aids weight loss by reducing appetite. In the article on diabetes in this section, we listed some twenty nutrients that help with insulin regulation. Most of these will also assist with weight loss. Some of the important insulin regulators appetite suppressants are:
- **Chromium**: This mineral has long had the reputation of helping weight loss, in the form of fat and replacing it with muscle by enhancing the action of insulin. It also assists in stabilizing blood sugar levels, increases metabolic rate, and tips energy levels.
- **Gymnema sylvestre**: This herb is reputed to make food taste less sweet so that the individual has less craving for it.
- **Magnesium**: Used in several ways during glucose metabolism, magnesium assists the body in maintaining blood sugar levels and is useful in combating fatigue as well.
- **Fenugreek**: This herb offers support for healthy glucose metabolism.

Hormone replacement therapy. As we grow older, our levels of certain hormones decrease. When we supplement and bring these up to the levels of youth, one of the changes we see is that the body's ratio of fat to muscle improves, often reaching the level we had when we were younger.
- **DHEA**: This hormone enhances metabolic efficiency. Low levels of DHEA are associated with obesity. Some researchers believe that it hinders the body's ability to store and produce fat.
- **Testosterone**: We see many obese men at the Wellness Centers who suffer from fatigue and low testosterone levels. Among the benefits they may receive from testosterone therapy are increased energy and increased muscle mass.
- **Human growth hormone**: Supplementing with HGH has been shown to change body composition, resulting in more muscle and less fat.

Diuretics. These make a contribution to weight loss by getting rid of excess fluid. The diuretic effect you get from eating asparagus can be obtained from asparagus capsules.

- Also important as a diuretic is **pyridoxal 5 phosphate,** a precursor to vitamin B-6. There are many herbal formulas that work as diuretics.

Probiotics or Intestinal Stabilizers. These aid in normalizing intestinal flora.
- The most effective are **acidophilus, glutamine, and fructo-oligosaccharides.**
- Two new enhancements are available at the Wellness Centers in the product called **Carbo-Control**.

Two other substances are worth mentioning. Lagerstroemia Speciosa L (brand name Glucosol) is a natural substance that has been used clinically, and I have found it to be quite successful. Studies show that it will enhance the transport of glucose into the body's cells. By improving glucose transport, it reduces glucose in the blood, lowers insulin resistance, increases energy, and burns fat. Phaseolamin is an extract of the white kidney bean. As an alpha-amylase inhibitor that blocks the breakdown of carbohydrates in the intestine, it therefore blocks ingested carbohydrates from getting into the bloodstream.

Chapter Nine
Insulin Resistance

Understanding Insulin Resistance

Are you among the millions of Americans who have tried low-fat diets many times yet failed to stick with them? Or perhaps you have lost weight, then gained it all back in a few months. There is a reason for these so-called failures, and it is not your lack of will power. The standard low-fat diet, which usually has a high carbohydrate content, is not right for most overweight people. The subject discussed in this chapter could shed some light on your problem. It is insulin resistance, and it is explained in depth here.

The majority of overweight people are insulin resistant. This means that their chronically high levels of insulin increase their cravings for carbohydrates and their body's tendency to store food energy in the form of fat. But when insulin resistant individuals go on a carbohydrate-regulated diet, their food cravings decrease markedly, and they are amazed at how easy it is to lose weight and to keep it off.

I understand insulin resistance and the accompanying carbohydrate addiction very well because I myself suffer from it. At one time I was 100 pounds overweight. I felt I had no control over my eating habits. I yearned for pasta at every meal and consumed large quantities of fruit (which people are surprised to learn, is very high in carbohydrates) and desserts. On the day I first read about insulin resistance and carbohydrate addiction a bell went off, and I recognized I was reading about myself. Using this diet I began to lose weight, and within eight months I lost the 100 pounds. I have kept it off ever since without a struggle. It's not because I have more will power than you do, but what I do have is the background and experience to research the topic of insulin resistance and to devise a weight reduction program based on scientific knowledge.

Insulin disorders are closely connected not only to people with overweight conditions, but also to other problems I see every day in my practice as a heart specialist; high blood pressure, high triglycerides, and diabetes, all of which put people at great risk for heart disease.

Insulin Resistance and Heart Disease

Until lately, the medical community has not recognized the crucial connection between insulin resistance and obesity and heart disease. About sixty percent of the patients I see in my practice at the Cardiovascular Wellness Centers have insulin-related problems. We now routinely give all patients glucose tolerance tests, which measure their insulin levels. In the past few years, new research has appeared in medical journals confirming much of what we have been saying for many years about insulin resistance and its related problems.

Research sponsored by the National Heart, Lung, and Blood Institute[50] in what is called a "landmark study of enormous importance," concluded that insulin resistance should be thought of as a new independent risk factor for heart disease. This means that high insulin levels alone can lead to heart disease in the absence of any other risk factors. Insulin problems commonly occur with other risk factors, including lipid disorders, hypertension, central obesity, glucose intolerance—a group of symptoms referred to as Syndrome X. "It would make more sense," says lead NIH investigator Dr. George Howard, "to try to correct the underlying disorder (insulin resistance) rather than separately treat each of the medical problems involved in Syndrome X." Dr. Howard elaborates, "some drugs that effectively lower blood pressure and lipid levels may actually increase insulin resistance and worsen long-term outcome."

Research published in 1998 from the Bogalusa Heart Study, a long-term epidemiological investigation of cardiovascular disease risk factors among children and young adults,[51] reveals the insidious destructiveness of insulin resistance. Insulin levels in children and young adults were measured and the subjects were followed over an eight-year period. Those subjects with high insulin levels had significantly more risk factors for heart disease, regardless of their age, race, or sex. Their parents were more likely to have a history of diabetes and hypertension. The children tended to have lipid abnormalities: elevated levels of cholesterol, triglycerides, VLDL (very low-density lipid) cholesterol and LDL cholesterol,

---

[50] "Diabetes Mellitus: A Major Risk Factor for Cardiovascular Disease," National Heart, Lung, and Blood Institute study, www.nhlbi.nih.gov/new/press/sep01-99.htm.
[51] The Bogalusa Heart Study (since 1972 out of Louisiana State University Medical Center) is the longest and most detailed study of children in the world. www.som.tulane.edu/cardiohealth/bog.htm.

along with lower levels of HDL or "good" cholesterol. They were likely to be overweight and suffer from high blood pressure.

In fact, the prevalence of obesity was 72 percent in subjects with persistently elevated insulin levels versus 2 percent in those with persistently low insulin levels. Hypertension was 2.5 times more common and lipid disorders three times more prevalent. Furthermore, those with high insulin levels had significant clustering of two or three risk factors, such as obesity/hypertension or hypertension/lipid disorders/obesity. These combinations, Syndrome X or the Deadly Quartet, are particularly potent risks for heart disease. The high insulin levels, and accompanying cardiovascular risk factors, didn't just go away or change as the children got older. Those participants with relatively high or low insulin levels retained such levels eight years later.

Researchers want to know how insulin works to cause these hazardous effects. Insulin appears to wreak its havoc by damaging the blood vessel walls. When this occurs, it initiates the accumulation of plaque, creating blockages, which lead to atherosclerosis and then heart disease. High insulin levels may also indirectly exacerbate the development of atherosclerosis. In the NHLBI study, men with insulin resistance were found to have greater thickness of the carotid artery wall then men without insulin resistance. Wall thickness of the carotid artery is an accepted way of predicting the extent of atherosclerosis in the rest of the circulatory system. Researchers continue to put together the pieces of the puzzle that begins with insulin resistance and ends with heart disease and death. As we add to this knowledge, we improve our methods of diagnosing and treating heart disease.

We may need to reevaluate many of our therapies for cardiovascular disease in view of recent findings about insulin resistance. A young man came in after hearing me say on my radio program that it's possible to eat too much fruit if you have an insulin problem. "I realized that although I'm eating what I've always thought was healthy, it could be the wrong thing," he said. And after an evaluation we found he indeed was insulin resistant and was eating too many carbohydrates in the form of potatoes and bread.

Most people who have insulin resistance, and the accompanying central abdominal obesity, lipid abnormalities, and high blood pressure need to be on a diet that is low in fat; but it is essential that it be carbohydrate-restricted as well. I recall another interesting patient recently who was slightly overweight. As is my standard procedure, I gave him a glucose tolerance test, and it revealed insulin resistance and a diabetic pattern.

The patient was terrified because his mother had suffered from diabetes. I put him on a strict modified-carbohydrate, low-fat diet. The next time I saw him, although he had lost only 12 pounds, he had a normal glucose tolerance test, indicating that the management of many cardiovascular and metabolic problems can be controlled with the right diet.

In view of what we now know about insulin resistance, physicians must reevaluate not only diet but also the pharmacologic therapy for these patients. Some drugs, such as beta-blockers and diuretics, can aggravate insulin resistance. Frequently prescribed for hypertension, these medications can also worsen the lipid profile and glucose control. On the other hand, the antihypertensive drug doxazosin (Cardura) was revealed to be very effective for managing hypertension because it counteracts the effects of insulin resistance. The newest findings on insulin resistance have far-reaching implications for the management of heart disease.

How Insulin Affects Heart Disease

What role does insulin play in heart disease? *Hyperinsulinemia,* which means an excess of insulin, is a hormonal imbalance that very often accompanies obesity, hypertension, high cholesterol and high triglycerides, atherosclerosis, stroke, adult-onset diabetes, and other diseases and conditions related to heart disease. Many people suffer from hyperinsulinemia and do not know it. In their book, Drs. Rachael and Richard Heller view hyperinsulinemia, which they call "Profactor-H," as the first and underlying disorder that not just accompanies but causes all of these other health problems. They believe that to get control of your health you must get control of your body's production of insulin.[52]

You may have heard of insulin only as a substance taken by diabetics, although our bodies make insulin, necessary to give us energy. Created in the pancreas, insulin is released into the blood after eating. It helps sugar get into the body's cells, where it is used as fuel for the cell's activities. We say a person is insulin resistant when the sugar does not move into the cells at a normal rate, but resists leaving the blood stream. This causes the pancreas to secrete even more insulin into the bloodstream, where it continues to circulate. If there is too much insulin in the bloodstream, it loses its effectiveness in performing its work. Probably 75 percent of overweight people are insulin resistant, experts estimate. It is

---

[52] Heller, Rachael and Richard, *The Carbohydrate Addict's Healthy for Life,* Dutton Plume, 1996.

the first step toward developing hypoglycemia, also known as glucose intolerance, and eventually diabetes.

Too much insulin has many other negative effects. For example, it stimulates cholesterol production in the liver. The cholesterol then flows through the bloodstream, encouraging the production of plaque in the blood vessels. The amount of adrenaline in the blood stream increases when someone has too much insulin. This raises the blood pressure and the heart rate. Insulin causes the kidneys to retain salt, further contributing to high blood pressure. An excess of insulin stimulates the body to produce and store fat and promotes the accumulation of fat in blood vessels, increasing the triglyceride level. Intense food cravings are created by too much insulin in the bloodstream, which leads to obesity, another major risk factor for heart disease.

The recognition of insulin's wide-ranging powers has led to the development of insulin-regulating diets. Carbohydrates are the villains for those people who have problems with insulin. Their blood sugar levels escalate shortly after they eat carbohydrates, creating irresistible food cravings and otherwise wreaking havoc in the body. In their book *Healthy for Life,* the Hellers advocate an eating plan that restricts carbohydrates entirely for two meals and allows them at a third. The Cardiovascular Wellness Centers also offers an insulin-regulating diet that is low in fat and allows some, but not many, carbohydrates throughout the day. These insulin-regulating diets have proven to be beneficial to many people who have not been able to lose weight on other diets.

How do you know if you have a problem with insulin? If you are overweight, chances are very good that you do. Here is part of the quiz offered by the Hellers to help make the determination. Do you find that maintaining a normal weight is a struggle? Do you often experience craving for carbohydrates such as sweets, bread, pasta, and potato chips? Are you tired in the middle of the afternoon? Are you hungry an hour or so after you finish eating? Do you have a tendency to retain fluid? Do you experience signs of low blood sugar (headache, weakness, irritability, sweats)?

If you suspect you have an insulin problem, you should ask your doctor for a glucose/insulin metabolism evaluation. Or, you can try an insulin-regulating diet to see if it gets rid of your symptoms and lets you succeed at losing weight. In addition to a modified carbohydrate diet, exercise is critical for the person with an insulin problem.

Carbohydrate addiction has become more of a problem as people move toward low-fat diets. It is very important to decrease the intake of fat but, for those who are insulin resistant, it is also necessary to avoid over consumption of starches and simple sugars in the form of bread, pasta, rice, potatoes, fruit and fruit juices, jams and jellies. It's a delicate balancing act, especially since many foods that carbohydrate addicts must avoid —such as fruit—are actually very healthful and necessary for those people who are not carbohydrate addicts.

At the Cardiovascular Wellness Centers, in addition to identifying patients who are carbohydrate sensitive and helping them control their hyperinsulinemia, we try to promote total body wellness through a multifaceted program that goes beyond diet. Our program utilizes metabolic enhancing nutrients, vitamins, removal of food sensitivities, and detoxification of the body. We find, for instance, that many patients have candida and what we will call intestinal dysbiosis (abnormal flora) that must be treated. These are all issues that relate to weight loss, diet, and nutrition and play key roles in achieving good health.

Diabetes & Heart Disease Are Inextricably Linked

Diabetics suffer a triple whammy when it comes to heart disease. Not only are they far more likely to have it than nondiabetics, but when they do develop heart disease, they very often do not experience any of the warning symptoms. As a result, their heart disease may remain undiagnosed until it has progressed dangerously. Or, their first symptom might be a heart attack—a particularly unfortunate circumstance because a heart attack is more likely to be fatal for them than for nondiabetics.

It is also not uncommon for diabetics to suffer a heart attack and not know it. This is because they may not feel the chest pain that is the usual warning sign. The diabetes can disturb the patients' nervous system, so that they do not perceive chest pain. Or sometimes a diabetic may feel chest pain, but attributes it to a glucose reaction. The doctor may discover that a heart attack has occurred when the patient undergoes an electrocardiogram at some later time. Diabetics must be aware of symptoms of heart attack other than chest pain: shortness of breath, sweatiness, unexplained nausea, vomiting, and fatigue. All of these can signal that their heart is not getting enough blood. Diabetics experiencing any of these warning signs should have a cardiac evaluation immediately.

Diabetes has doubled in the last 20 years, a factor attributed to an aging, increasingly sedentary, and overweight population. The risk factors for both heart disease and diabetes are the same, and they multiply the harmful effects of each other.

Common risk factors that diabetics and heart patients share are listed below:

Insulin resistance. The cluster of risk factors called Syndrome X that goes with insulin resistance precede the onset of diabetes and predict its occurrence. When insulin resistance goes unchecked, glucose intolerance is likely to develop. With glucose intolerance, the risk of progression to diabetes is 2-5 percent a year.

Hypertension. Diabetes also increases all the harmful effects of high blood pressure. Most people with hypertension experience it only during waking hours. As they sleep, their system gets rest. Not with diabetics. Their blood pressure is high 24 hours a day, putting a continual strain on the arteries and the heart.

Obesity. Just as the risk for heart disease increases with gaining weight, the risk for diabetes doubles in the mildly obese, is five times greater for the moderately obese, and ten times greater in the severely obese. Furthermore, both groups of patients are likely to have a specific type of obesity, with their weight concentrated in the abdomen. This abdominal fat is of a different type from fat elsewhere on the body. It creates a very high influx of fatty acids into the liver. These cannot be metabolized and result in hypertriglyceridernia.

Lipid abnormalities. Diabetics are likely to have the lipid abnormalities that cause heart disease. These include the dangerous pattern of small, dense LDL cholesterol, high triglycerides, and low levels of the beneficial HDL cholesterol.

Physical inactivity. A sedentary lifestyle promotes heart disease and diabetes. Low intensity, prolonged exercise will substantially reduce insulin levels, thus lowering the risk of both diseases.

Diabetics should be aware of how inextricably their disease is linked to heart disease, know the warning signs of heart disease, and treat the shared risk factors. When I discuss diabetes on the radio show, as I frequently do, I hope that people who consider themselves nondiabetics are paying attention. The incidence of undiagnosed diabetes is astronomical. There is currently an epidemic of obesity in the United States, and a great number of overweight people are getting Type 2 Diabetes—also known as adult onset diabetes. If they are not overt diabetics, they often are glucose intolerant or pre-diabetic. These patients fall into the same genetic characteristic group, and they should heed many of the things we talk about for management of diabetes. In my practice, I stress the importance of the glucose tolerance test. A week does not go by that I don't discover a few cases of diabetes by this test, as well as many cases of glucose intolerance. I find diabetes in individuals who have been followed by their regular doctor for years and years, yet their diabetes has not been detected because they have not been given this test.

Diabetics can have a heart attack without knowing it. We call this silent ischemia, and recently researchers have discovered that silent ischemia occurs much more frequently than they had thought, often in non-diabetics as well. Many diabetics are rushed to the emergency room with what they think are uncontrolled diabetic complications, such as high blood sugar or gastrointestinal upset, and it turns out to be a heart attack. The major symptoms of diabetes are increased fatigue, frequent urination, and inability to lose weight because of improper diet, which results in progressive diabetic complications. Anyone who has these symptoms or risk factors for diabetes should be tested for the disease.

Solving the Diet Dilemma

As carbohydrate-restricted diets become more popular, controversy rages about what is the proper diet for the management of heart disease, weight loss, and good nutrition. In a recent article called "Garbo-phobia," in the July/August issue of the newsletter of Science in the Public Interest, writer Bonnie Liebman denigrates and discounts many of the well-proven and documented advantages of a high protein, restricted carbohydrate, insulin-regulating diet.[53] While most of her criticism is aimed at Barry Sears's book *The Zone*, she also attacks other popular diets: *Thin for Life* and *Protein Power*.[54]

All this adds to the confusion about the proper diet. Not too many years ago, health experts urged everyone to slash the fat content of their diet in order to lose weight, lower their cholesterol, and avoid atherosclerosis. So people loaded up on carbohydrates in the form of pasta, bread, rice, potatoes, fruit, and fruit juices. They gobbled up low-fat brownies and all the other "diet" products that filled the supermarket shelves. They hailed low-fat dieting as the panacea for weight loss and good health. It soon became clear, however, that people were not losing

---

[53] Liebmann, Bonnie, Director of Nutrition for the Center for Science in the Public Interest, a voluntary advocacy group for nutrition and food safety, located in Washington DC, www.scpinet.org.
[54] Sears, Dr. Barry, *The Zone: A Dietary Roadmap*, HarperCollins, 1995; Fletcher, Anne F., *Thin for Life*, HarperCollins 1994; Eades, Michael and Mary, *Protein Power*, Bantam Books, 1996.

weight; a government report appeared saying that in the last decade the percentage of overweight Americans increased from 25 percent of the population to 33 percent. Studies showed that about 95 percent of people who went on a diet and lost weight gained it all back in five years. The low-fat diet might be right in theory (without question it was necessary to lower cholesterol and fight atherosclerosis) but in practice few people were able to take off weight and keep it off.

Then articles began to appear with frequency in the medical journals from researchers who found that many overweight people (as many of 75 percent of them) suffered from a condition called insulin resistance. For a number of reasons, these people had too much insulin in their blood, and they were at high risk for developing what came to be known as Syndrome X—the aforementioned cluster of factors that included obesity, high blood pressure, high triglycerides, and glucose intolerance. Scientists had known for years that these conditions occur together, and they now began to suspect that insulin resistance was causing the other conditions. For these people with insulin resistance, a diet high in carbohydrates made their bodies respond with intense cravings for more carbohydrates and with weight gain. These, in turn, made the insulin resistance worse and increased their risk factors for heart disease.

Previously discussed in this book, I laid out the inexorable way in which a high carbohydrate diet could lead to heart disease for some people. More and more books on low carbohydrate dieting came on the market. The reason for their popularity was simple; for many people, they worked. Those who were insulin resistant found that for the first time they had a diet they could stick to and their intense cravings for food became a thing of the past. This now brings us to several questions that have fueled the controversy:

1. Is a carbohydrate-restricted diet right for everyone? One pair of eyeglasses does not fit all. A carbohydrate-restricted diet is correct for those people who are insulin resistant. We have to identify them and be sure their diet is not only carbohydrate restricted, but also high in protein and low in fat.
2. Those individuals who are on carbohydrate-restricted diets must maintain a low fat intake as well. A low-fat diet is essential for everyone. Those fats that we do consume should be monounsaturated. Saturated fat should be avoided as much as possible. One reason for the controversy surrounding carbohydrate-restricted diets is that some of them do not limit fat, nor even saturated fat. They allow bacon and

eggs for breakfast and all the steak you can eat for dinner. These diets often bring about weight loss, but they are not good for your heart health.

3. Vegetables and a certain amount of fruit are extremely important. Because some vegetables and most fruit are high in carbohydrates, people on very low carbohydrate diets have to cut out too much of these items. In my experience, these dieters tend to rebound intensively to a very high fat diet.

4. The last important point: those who are not insulin resistant do well on a Mediterranean-type diet, which advocates very little meat, generous amounts of fruits and vegetables, monounsaturated fats such as olive and canola oil, and plenty of bread, pasta, rice, other grains, and potatoes.

The importance of low-fat dieting and the relationship between insulin resistance, obesity and risk factors for heart disease are all well documented in the medical literature. These scientific conclusions—unlike anecdotal stories that we hear from people promoting some nutritional theories—rely on reviewing angiograms and other hard evidence, not just wishing that things would get better.

I have several other caveats. In my practice, I treat all patients as individuals in terms of the kind and intensity of diet, drug therapy, and vitamin programs, depending on the severity of their disease. A patient with severe angina or peripheral vascular disease will get a much more intensive program than a patient coming in for weight loss and heart disease prevention. In my waiting room two heart patients began exchanging information about their successful dieting, and each was quite surprised about my recommendations, because I had put one on a vegetarian diet and the other on a moderate carbohydrate, high protein, low-fat diet. Weight loss and good nutrition are complex matters. As scientific research progresses we find different ways to help different patients. There is no panacea that can guarantee weight loss and good health to all. And one size does not fit all.

Carbohydrate Addiction: Not Just a Weight Problem

Many patients who come to my centers are carbohydrate addicts. They suffer from hunger all the time and crave pasta, bread, and sweets. They have tried and failed at many diets. They may visit the Wellness Centers for treatment of their overweight condition or for one of the several disorders that goes along with carbohydrate addiction. The carbohydrate addict can usually be spotted immediately. He or she not only is overweight, but also carries the weight in the abdominal area. This is what doctors call central abdominal obesity, which is simply a fat stomach.

It's also likely that carbohydrate addicts will have another medical condition: high blood pressure. And because they cannot lose weight, their hypertension usually gets worse with age. If we check the carbohydrate addict's total cholesterol level, it may not be elevated. But a closer look will reveal a dangerous lipid pattern. The triglyceride level will be high and the HDL (or beneficial cholesterol) will be low. In addition, many of these patients are suffering from diabetes, often undiagnosed by their family doctors.

All these conditions—carbohydrate addiction, central abdominal obesity, hypertension, high triglycerides, low HDL, diabetes or a pre-diabetic condition—are a package deal. If a person has one, he or she is at risk for acquiring the others. Together they are known as Syndrome X, and they put an individual at high risk for developing atherosclerosis and heart disease. The underlying condition that experts believe contributes to all of these disorders is the inability of the body to process insulin properly, called insulin resistance or hyperinsulinemia. Chronically high levels of insulin increase the craving for carbohydrates. Dr. Rachael Heller tells us, "the enjoyment of carbohydrate rich food and the body's tendency to store food energy in the form of fat, causes carbohydrate addicts to struggle to control their eating, without realizing that their bodies are fighting them by giving overpowering signals to eat, store food as fat, and to set their bodies up for progressive health problems."[55]

For carbohydrate addicts, losing weight is not the only problem. They must be alert to all the accompanying medical disorders that go with their carbohydrate addiction. Chances are good that carbohydrate addicts will have to deal with some or all of these conditions at some point in their lives. Getting on an insulin-regulating diet is the first step the carbohydrate addict must take. It will not only promote weight loss, but will improve the accompanying disorders. In addition, a vitamin program is necessary to get insulin under control. And don't forget about exercise; it's important

---

[55] Heller, Rachael and Richard, *The Carbohydrate Addict's Lifespan Program,* Dutton Plume, 2001.

in regulating insulin. Resistance-type exercises, such as those involving weights, are particularly good at combating visceral obesity.

Carbohydrate Addict's Quiz®

Are You a Carbohydrate Addict? (Answer Yes or No.)

1. After eating a full breakfast, do you get hungrier before it's time for lunch than if you had skipped breakfast altogether?
2. Do you get very tired after eating a large meal?
3. Do you often get tired and/or hungry in the afternoon?
4. Once you start to eat sweets, snack foods, or starches, do you have a difficult time stopping?
5. Have you been on diet after diet, only to regain all the weight that you lose (or more)?
6. Does stress, boredom, or tiredness make you want to eat?
7. Do you sometimes feel that you aren't satisfied even though you have just finished a meal?
8. Do you find it harder to take off weight and keep it off with each passing year?
9. Do you drink fruit juice, sports drinks, or soda (diet or regular) several times each day?
10. Do you take insulin, female replacement hormones, birth control pills, medication for high blood pressure or cholesterol problems, or regularly use chewable antacid tablets?

Scoring: Count your *yes* answers.

0-1: If you answered *yes* to fewer than two questions, you are probably not carbo-addicted. Therefore, any weight or health problems that you may have are probably not related to excess levels of insulin.

2-3: If you answered *yes* to two questions, you are probably mildly carbohydrate-addicted. You may be tempted to eat carbohydrate rich food sometimes, but usually you are able to control this impulse.

4-6: If you answered *yes* to four, five, or six questions, it is likely that you have a moderate carbohydrate addiction that has gone undiagnosed and untreated. You may be able to control your cravings for food some of the time, but when you are tired or stressed or ill, your ability to control your eating disappears. You probably have recurring concerns about your weight and your eating habits.

7-10: If you answered *yes* to seven or more questions, you probably have a severe carbohydrate addiction that may be greatly affecting your weight, health, and life. You experience recurring hunger and food cravings, which can sometimes be overwhelming. You may have mood swings and may experience physical symptoms such as fatigue, nervousness or irritability.[56]

Although I write often about diets, including weight loss programs and diets for heart disease, I feel the topic must constantly be revisited and accentuated. Avoiding carbohydrates seem to be such an important aspect of good health. My patients who have said they were quite surprised when I mentioned on my radio program that I do indeed eat Napoleons and other desserts. I have found that in order to be compliant with a diet, most people (including myself) must feel there is room for alternative types of eating. The complete removal of sugar from a normal person's diet is absolutely ridiculous. Even individuals with weight problems using the Carbohydrate Addict's program have been able to successfully lose weight while eating desserts. I myself have had to deal with a major weight problem—having been 100 pounds overweight at one point in my life. I now follow the Carbohydrate Addict's program and I often enjoy dessert.

Of course, for those with diabetes and those on insulin, the use of sugar has to be considered on an individual basis. I would not recommend apple pie and ice cream for someone with severe glucose problems. The obesity problems in this country are staggering, and they are getting more serious each year. Both the medical profession and the weight loss industry have failed to help people find solutions to overweight conditions. A recent report indicates that the majority of obese individuals are not on any kind of diet, having given up all hope of ever losing weight. This high failure rate makes me think we must be more lenient and look for long-term goals. Individuals should lose weight slowly over a long period of time. They should be able to have some enjoyment from food and at the same time achieve what is called metabolic fitness.

---

[56] *1997®, The Carbohydrate Addict's Quiz is a registered trademark of Dr. Richard and Rachael Heller. All rights reserved. Reproduction in part or whole, including but not limited to reproduction, transmission, modification, distribution, and republication, without the prior written permission of Dr. Richard and Rachael is strictly prohibited. (Used with permission.)*

time. They should be able to have some enjoyment from food and at the same time achieve what is called metabolic fitness.

In Dieting, One Size Does Not Fit All

I had a young patient in my office recently who was very thin and exercised a lot. He had heard me talk on the radio about the importance of a diet that restricts carbohydrates. He was confused about what kind of eating program he should be on to maintain good health. When I told him what he needed was a high-carbohydrate, low-fat diet, he was astonished. Wasn't Dr. Vagnini the low-carb advocate? What this patient didn't hear was something I very often reiterate: one diet does not fit all. A carbohydrate-restricted diet is the correct one for most overweight people because they very likely are insulin resistant.

More and more research is appearing to indicate the connection between insulin, overweight conditions and heart disease. A carbohydrate-restricting diet controls insulin levels. The overweight people I see in my office are over consuming carbohydrates. When they hear that they will have to cut back, they are devastated because they believe that they will have nothing to eat that they like. Indeed, almost no one ever has a craving for lettuce or celery. Most of the foods we crave are carbohydrates, whether desserts or potato chips or a big bowl of pasta.

Let's review the list of carbohydrates. While most people think of bread, pasta, rice, potatoes, cereal, and desserts, in fact, many vegetables are high in carbohydrates, including corn, peas, beans (except green beans), beets, sweet potatoes, and carrots. And many people are surprised to learn that on a carbohydrate-restricted diet, they must cut back on fruits and fruit juices, which are high in carbohydrates. Usually, my weight-loss patients have just one fruit a day, preferably an apple or pear.

We work with patients on an individual basis, and we hesitate to give one diet to everyone. Those who are not overweight and want to prevent or curtail heart disease should probably be on a standard low-fat diet, such as the one recommended by the American Heart Association. Younger more active patients can consume more carbohydrates than older sedentary patients. But those who are overweight with abdominal obesity, or high blood pressure, glucose intolerance, or diabetes—or who have any combination of those characteristics—almost certainly have an insulin problem, therefore their carbohydrate intake must be restricted. We often find yeast (candida) in patients who are over consuming carbohydrates, which sets them up for a range of additional problems. They must not only drastically reduce their carbohydrates but must go on a program of detoxification.

Many of the carbohydrate-restricted diets give a daily carbohydrate allowance of usually 25-30 grams. I find that this confuses people. At the Wellness Centers, we focus on size and number of portions a day. For example, someone who is overweight and sedentary but without serious health problems would be moderately restricted. He or she could have a carbohydrate intake in the course of a day that included a half cup of brown rice, two slices of whole grain bread, and perhaps a small amount (1/4 cup) of oatmeal for breakfast. A typical dinner would consist of crudités, salad, fish, or fowl, two low-carbohydrate vegetables, a small carbohydrate portion, and possibly, a sensible dessert. But we do not put people on a hard and fast diet. We monitor and counsel our patients continuously. As a patient loses weight or begins to exercise more, or shows other improvements, we may allow larger portions of rice, an occasional dish of pasta, or a baked potato. We try to achieve an eating program that a person can follow for a lifetime. If it is too restrictive, the patient will not be able to stay on it for a long time.

Breakfast is particularly difficult for people who are trying to cut their carbohydrate intake. Conscientious dieters may have given up the high fat breakfast of fried eggs and bacon and replaced it with a supposedly healthful morning meal of cereal, bananas, fruit juice, and milk, all of which are carbohydrates! While this is a perfectly healthy meal for someone who is not overweight and insulin resistant, for those who are, such a meal is dangerous, and it sets in motion a day of craving for more and more carbohydrates. We recommend a breakfast of egg whites or Eggbeaters, perhaps with vegetables or a small amount of oatmeal.

One reason people are confused about carbohydrate-restricted diets is that many fruits and some vegetables are not included in it. From all they read in reputable sources, these are the keystones of a healthy diet. For those individuals who are not insulin resistant, this is indeed true. For many people, especially those who can't come to the Wellness Centers, we suggest reading the Heller's book, *The Carbohydrate Addict's Healthy for Life*,[57] which restricts the frequency of carbohydrate intake rather than the amount. Many people are very successful with this diet, which, like our own program, (found at the end of this section) offers an eating plan for life.

---

[57]Heller, Rachael and Richard, *The Carbohydrate Addict's Healthy for Life*, Dutton Plume, 1996.

Finding the Right Insulin-Regulating Diet

By taking the carbohydrate addict's test (see previous section), you can determine whether a carbohydrate-restricted diet is for you. Other carbohydrate-restricted diets are available, however, and patients frequently ask us about the differences among them. Known as low-carb diets (although many of them would more accurately be called modified-carbohydrate diets), these eating plans take the approach that chronically high levels of insulin increase the craving for carbohydrates and the body's tendency to store food energy in the form of fat.

These high insulin levels exist in many overweight people and are exacerbated by a high intake of carbohydrate-rich food. The diets attempt to regulate insulin production by regulating carbohydrate intake, but each one approaches this issue in a different way. Counting calories is generally not a part of these diets. We recommend the Hellers' program, because many people are successful with it. It is easy to follow and easy to stay on indefinitely. It lowers insulin levels by changing the frequency of carbohydrate intake as opposed to controlling the amount of carbohydrates. This eating plan calls for two meals a day that are very low in carbohydrates, and then a third meal, called the "reward meal" during which dieters can eat carbohydrates and have almost anything else they want. We find that dieters are more successful if they know that they can have one meal a day in which they are not limited, and during which they can even have dessert. The diet can be undertaken in a low fat or vegetarian version. It requires no measuring or counting calories.

Another popular eating program is set forth in the book *The Zone* by Dr. Barry Sears. Dr. Sears considers his diet to be carbohydrate moderate, protein adequate, and low fat.[58] To control the body's insulin level, his main rule is that dieters keep a beneficial ratio of protein to carbohydrate every time they eat. The diet proportions are 40/30/30 (carb/fat/protein), a combination that, he says, keeps the insulin level in a "tight zone"—not too high and not too low, but where optimal performance is achieved. It calls for large servings of fruits and vegetables. Critics of the Zone diet say it can be too complicated to figure out these proportions, when, for instance, dealing with a slice of pizza and a salad.

Most people first heard of low carbohydrate dieting from Dr. Robert Atkins, whose original diet was published two decades ago and whose

---

[58] Sears, Dr. Barry, *The Zone: A Dietary Roadmap*, HarperCollins, 1995.

140

recent book the *New Diet Revolution*[57] is widely used.[59] On this diet, carbohydrates are so restricted as to be almost completely banished from every meal. This lack of carbohydrates puts the dieter in a state called "ketosis." In ketosis, because the body is not getting any carbohydrates, the individual uses up his store of glycogen or blood sugar, and the body goes into a fat burning mode in order to fuel the bodily functions. Dr. Atkins believes this is desirable, but many other experts think it is unhealthy. They point out that the body goes into ketosis from diabetes or starvation. Although his critics have also said his diet is high in fat, he claims it is not, that the dieter will eat less fat that on an ordinary diet. We do not use this diet at the Cardiovascular Wellness Centers because, while it may lower cholesterol and high triglycerides in some patients, the LDLs, which are atherogenic, do not go down. Carbohydrate-restricted diets are not for everyone, but for those individuals who fit the profile of a carbohydrate addict, this type of eating program can be the key to lifelong weight control.

Although the Cardiovascular Wellness Centers started out dealing with heart disease, it soon became apparent that most of my patients with high blood pressure, diabetes, heart attack, stroke, high cholesterol, and high triglycerides all required dietary adjustment, and many of these individuals were overweight as well. I decided to make weight reduction my subspecialty. I became a member of the American Society of Bariatric Physicians and brought Maria Santoro on staff as the dietitian. We now have a very successful weight reduction program, and much of my practice is dedicated to helping my patients make dietary changes both for weight loss and good health.

It is especially important to assist individuals in losing weight through dietary changes in view of recent warnings of severe complications from using some of the most widely prescribed drug therapies for weight loss. Fen-phen appears to cause valvular heart disease in some people, according to findings from the Mayo Clinic. I have recommended that all my patients taking this type of drug therapy for weight loss discontinue it.

---

[59] Atkins, Dr. Robert C., *Dr. Atkins' New Diet Revolution*, Morrow, William & Co, 2001.

Changing Concepts of Weight Loss

Toward the end of 2001, Dr. David Satcher, Surgeon General of the United States, issued a report in which he announced that our nation is currently experiencing an epidemic of obesity. Among the shocking statistics: 61 percent of American adults and 13 percent of our children are overweight. The vast majority—more than 95 percent of Americans—who take off weight, gain it all back within five years. Traditional solutions to the problem of being overweight, such as low-fat diets and exercise, have, for the most part, not worked. I alerted readers to the news that there are indications that the most popular drug therapy for weight loss, the combination of *fenfluramine* and *phentermine*, known as *fen phen* was associated with some cases of valvular heart disease. For physicians who want to assist patients in losing weight and for the obese patients themselves, this news was a blow. It has been only recently that drugs to help patients lose weight have become respectable again. They were out of favor after the backlash against amphetamines in the 1970s. It was thought that fen phen, marketed under the name of Redux, might open a new era of weight control in which physicians would be able to give their patients a significant tool that could make a difference when used in conjunction with a program of diet and exercise. But, in 1997, the FDA, acting on evidence regarding significant side effects associated with fen phen, asked the manufacturers to withdraw it from the marketplace.

First, it does not mean that these drugs will never be used. Fen phen and Redux are not, and never were, intended for people who want to lose a quick ten pounds before their class reunion. They are for patients who are severely obese, and doctors, if they prescribe them at all, must use great caution balancing the risk of a patient remaining overweight against the risk that weight-loss medication may present. If patients continue to use the drugs, they should be aware of the hazards and should be carefully monitored by their physician. Patients who have been taking fen phen are advised to consult with their physician. Stopping the drug abruptly may result in certain health hazards. Meanwhile, the search for a safe and effective weight loss drug continues. Where does this leave those overweight people who have failed on one diet after another? The search for a safe and effective weight loss drug continues. *Orlistat*, the first of a new class called lipase inhibitors, in 1997 was recommended for approval by a committee within the FDA as a long-term treatment for obesity. It is marketed under the name, *Xenical*. This drug acts in the gastrointestinal tract to block the absorption of fat by 30 percent. Patients in a one-year clinical trial, lost approximately 10 percent of their body weight after taking Xenical along with following a moderately reduced caloric protocol. They had significant reductions in total and LDL cholesterol, blood pressures, and improvements in glucose and insulin levels. The most common side effects of the drug were gastrointestinal, and these generally disappeared in time. Several other drugs are currently in clinical trials, and within the next few years doctors and patients will have an array of choices.

For those who are severely overweight (more than 100 pounds) there is another option: weight loss-surgery. This is for the person whose health is threatened by obesity and who has tried everything else, many times. Surgery to treat severe obesity involves reducing the size of the stomach so that it holds much less food. The patient will very quickly feel full and further eating will bring on nausea and vomiting. Patients who have the surgery on average lose about 40 percent of their excess weight. In addition to the surgery, they must follow a lifetime program of diet, exercise, and vitamins. Doctors require that the patient have the ability to remain committed to a long-term program of weight loss. The goal of weight-loss surgery is not cosmetic, but it is meant to improve health conditions that have become life threatening, such as advanced cardiovascular disease, degenerative arthritis, diabetes, and very high blood pressure. Weight loss surgery may seem an extreme measure, but some people are desperate. Obesity is a persistent physical condition of multifactorial origin that requires lifelong treatment. It is a real disease, often genetically based. Those patients who have dieted unsuccessfully many times should find a doctor who is trained to deal with obesity.

Weight loss is constantly in the news. There is increasing interest in our Wellness Newsletter because readers feel we give good directions for managing weight. Don't forget; the goal of weight loss is good health and metabolic fitness. This means that the person should try to reach not the weight of the trendiest supermodel, but the weight that will normalize his or her blood sugar, insulin level, cholesterol, triglycerides, and blood pressure. We have discussed many aspects of weight reduction: diets, drugs, exercise, vitamins, and, even surgery. The most important step in being successful at weight reduction is to go to a center that is associated with the American Society of Bariatricians. Bariatrics is the study of weight loss. A physician who has a subspecialty in bariatrics, as I do, will have up-to-date information on how to help you and will have a staff that is knowledgeable and dedicated to the goal of assisting patients in losing weight.

The second most important element that will enable the individual to achieve weight-loss success is commitment. I have seen people religiously come back to the Wellness Centers time after time. They stick to their program, and they gradually reach a healthy weight. Once you have had a stroke or manifest the complications of diabetes it's too late. You will say to yourself, "why didn't I make that commitment?" The investment of time and effort pays off. You must try to find a way to make this commitment to change your behavior and your attitude. You need more than the superficial goal of fitting into a new outfit. Stay healthy for your children and grandchildren and for your own longevity.

Obesity Problems Start at an Early Age

Although we realize that children are unlikely to be reading this book, we are addressing the topic of children and obesity because most of our readers are parents or grandparents. We want to alert them to the fact that childhood obesity has become a dangerous national epidemic, and adults must take a role in guiding children toward good nutritional habits and weight loss. First of all, few children eat properly. A study in the *Journal of Pediatrics* that tracked the food intake of over 3,000 children, revealed that only one percent of them were meeting the Food Guide Pyramid recommendation for proper nutrition.[60] Sixteen percent of them did not meet national recommendations in any category of food. Children's diets have far too much fat and sugar.

From time to time, I have interviewed Rachael and Richard Heller on my radio program. They explained how easy it is for certain children to have excessive amounts of sugars, sweets and carbohydrates.[61] This often occurs because of overindulgence in fruit juice, breakfast cereal, and sugary snacks. This leads not only to weight problems but also emotional instability, learning disabilities, fatigue, and behavioral problems. Even if the children don't gain weight now, they will develop weight problems in later life. This is an important book that everyone with children and grandchildren must read, whether or not their kids have weight problems. Two other important investigations of childhood obesity have appeared recently. The *New England Journal of Medicine* has reported that kids

---

[60] Muñoz, Kathryn A. , et al., *Food Intakes of US Children and Adolescents Compared With Recommendations,* Pediatrics, September 1997.
[61] Heller, Rachael and Richard , *Carbohydrate-Addicted Kids,* Harper Trade, 1998.

with obese parents have a much greater likelihood of becoming obese.[62] Parental obesity more than doubles a child's risk of adult obesity. Furthermore, if the child is overweight and has overweight parents, the likelihood of becoming an obese adult is very great. I think this is due not only to genetics but also to the type of diet the children are given.

Overweight parents pass on their poor eating habits to their children. Because overweight has a genetic component, we should not take that to mean there is nothing we can do about it. A woman phoned my radio program recently and said she was obese because it was inherited, and she believed I was unfair and cruel to castigate people for being overweight when there is nothing they can do about it. When I weighed 300 pounds, I agreed with her. I thought it was my genetic destiny, because I come from a family with a lot of obese people. But I eventually discovered that I did have control over my weight, and I modified my diet and lost a hundred pounds. It is too easy to use the genetic excuse—both for yourself and your kids. If there is a genetic predisposition to being overweight in your family, it is all the more important to see to it that your children eat properly and get regular exercise. Above all, don't make the mistake of thinking children will outgrow their weight problems.

Finally, in a presentation at an American Heart Association meeting,[61] Dr. Alan Sinaiko of the University of Minnesota Medical School reported he discovered a significant relationship between insulin resistance in pre-teens and teenagers, especially boys, relating to major factors for heart disease risk in later life.[63] Using a sophisticated research tool called the insulin clamp, he found a high incidence of insulin resistance among teenagers, which we know indicates that the cells of the body take up glucose less efficiently than normal. Boys who showed insulin resistance also had higher blood levels of "bad" (LDL) cholesterol and higher blood pressure. (The correlation was less significant in girls). Obese children were more likely to have this problem, but it appeared in children who were not overweight as well. Kids usually don't have heart attacks or strokes, but this subtle abnormality in the way they react to insulin may identify early those facing increased risks in adulthood of heart attack, stroke, hypertension, overweight, diabetes, and other health problems.

---

[62] Rocchini, A.P., *Childhood Obesity and a Diabetes Epidemic*, New England Journal of Medicine, March 14, 2002.

[63] Ellis, Lisa, "Early Signs Of Cardiovascular Disease Seen In Adolescence," Inteli-Health News Service, September 25, 2001, www.intelihealth.com.

What all this indicates is that poor nutrition and overweight conditions in childhood can set kids on a path that leads to a lifetime of poor health. It can create emotional and behavioral problems. It is key to later heart disease. Children who are overweight is a condition that should not be taken lightly. I gave a talk on heart disease to my daughter Grace's fifth grade class. I told them that management of heart problems begins in youth and that the three most important elements are proper diet, weight control, and regular exercise. Fifth grade is not too early to make children themselves aware of the importance of what they eat. But parents and grandparents must provide the guidance toward a healthy adulthood through proper nutrition.

Beyond Dieting

I have focused on losing weight primarily by choosing the right diet. But there are other important aspects to this topic, and in this section I want to discuss the critical components of successful weight loss in addition to the diet program.

1. **Get motivated.** Motivation is key to successful weight loss. You must find the inspiration to do the hard work and make the commitment to dropping pounds. People report a variety of motivations, such as wanting to look good for their daughter's wedding or desiring to live a long life for their grandchildren. But you must discover your own motivation and you must do it now. As you get older your health will deteriorate if you are overweight: you will be at much greater risk for heart disease, hypertension, diabetes, and a host of other diseases. And you must lose weight now, because as you get older it becomes more difficult.

2. **Establish goals.** In her newsletter column, Maria Santoro has explained how to set short-term and long-term weight loss goals. Keep in mind when setting your personal goals that obese people do not do well if they lose too much weight or lose it too rapidly. If you are obese, your goal should be to attain metabolic fitness. This is the weight that will make you feel good, at which your blood pressure, glucose levels, cholesterol, and other lipid levels are under control.

3. **Enhance energy.** I find that many overweight patients are very fatigued most of the time, and this condition must be addressed. Without

146

energy they are likely to spend their time in front of the television or napping, rather than living a vigorous active life that would contribute to weight loss. They are likely to be apathetic, unable to make the effort they need to lose weight. We have nutrients that will enhance energy. My patients have had particular success with Coenzyme Q10 and lipoic acid or a formulation called CoQ10Plus.

4. **Intestinal toxicity.** Often the fatigue that overweight people experience, is due to intestinal toxicity: yeast, candida, or parasites. Many have toxicity from chemicals held in the fatty tissue of their bodies, or they have chronic viral syndrome, which also requires nutritional therapy. So it's important to first enhance energy, then detoxify the systems. Certain nutrients will accomplish that.

5. **Regulate hormones.** DHEA, the hormone that manufactures the sex hormones, is an adjunct therapy for weight loss. In women, the lack of progesterone can be a problem and replacement of it with transcutaneous progesterone cream helps women lose weight. In men with low testosterone levels, it may be important to replace this male sex hormone. Another substance to consider is called growth hormone, which I believe will eventually be the superstar weight-loss hormone.

6. **Use other nutritional therapies.** High potency multivitamins and antioxidants are indispensable for anyone losing weight. I have reported on success of the formulation *Carbo Stable* in regulating glucose levels. Essential oils are very important, as are the two newest supplements we are using at the Wellness Centers, *pyruvate/DHA and CLA (conjugated linoleic acid).*

7. **Embark on an exercise program.** Physical activity is a fundamental part of losing weight. It is difficult to give a general prescription because each individual needs a different exercise program, depending on his or her level of fitness, age, etc. But at a minimum, patients should be on a regular walking program of thirty minutes per day, most days of the week. In addition, resistance training exercise with dumbbells is essential, particularly for older patients, because it not only builds up muscles, it also improves insulin resistance.

Of course, at the Cardiovascular Wellness Centers the real secret weapon to fighting obesity is Maria Santoro, our nutritionist who assists

147

patients in putting together the whole weight-loss package. She is one of the leading medical nutritionists in the country. In addition to offering food counseling, she is very knowledgeable about exercise and an expert in the nutritional management of obesity and diabetes. Making a qualified nutritionist part of your program is a key to your success.

Summing Up

When health conscious people embrace low fat cooking, they tend to cut back on the amount of meat they eat and substitute pasta and other carbohydrates for it. What's wrong with eating more pasta, bread, rice, and potatoes? Plenty, if you are among the estimated 25 percent of the population that is considered insulin-resistant. "Insulin resistance" will become the buzz words in the diet and nutrition fields in the coming years. For people with this condition, eating carbohydrates creates a craving for more carbohydrates. They gain weight and have difficulty losing it. It is estimated that 95 percent of overweight people are insulin resistant.

A growing number of researchers are now acknowledging that one of the reasons so many diets fail (and we know that 95 percent of dieters gain back whatever weight they have lost within five years) is that we are not acknowledging the role of insulin in our diets. Persons who are insulin resistant have an imbalance in their body's levels of this hormone. When they eat carbohydrates more insulin than necessary is released into the blood. Too much insulin in the blood results in increased hunger and cravings for carbohydrate rich food, increased fat storage in fat cells, and a decreased ability to remove fat from fat cells.

But the weight problems of insulin-resistant people are not the worst of it. Insulin resistance may set up a whole syndrome of serious health problems that put those who have this condition at highest risk for heart disease. Everyone who is overweight should have a glucose/insulin metabolism evaluation.

Syndrome X

Scientists have noted that insulin resistance is usually accompanied by high blood pressure, cholesterol abnormalities, high blood sugar, diabetes or a prediabetic condition, and central abdominal obesity. This group of disorders has been christened Syndrome X, and people with the syndrome are the most likely to have heart attacks. Scientists have know for years that these disorders occur together, but only recently have they come to believe that it may be insulin resistance that causes the accompanying conditions. In the new guidelines published in May 2001 by the National Cholesterol Education Program of the NIH, it is referred to as the "metabolic syndrome."

Fighting Insulin Resistance

But here is the good news. There are ways to reduce insulin resistance. Weight loss is the most important method of controlling the condition, and this should be done through a low-fat, low-carbohydrate, high-protein diet. This means that in addition to the usual restrictions of a low-fat diet, one must also greatly limit the intake of sugar and starches. Foods that should be de-accentuated, are rice, pasta, potatoes, cereal, corn, peas, sweet potatoes, desserts, dairy products, meats, and fruit with a high sugar content. Items that are somewhat limited are bread and grains. It may at first glance seem as if there's nothing you can eat, but that is not the case. It does mean a diet of chicken, turkey, fish, non-starchy vegetables, legumes, and limited grains. For those who are insulin resistant, the diet is usually not that difficult to follow because they no longer have the food cravings they have experienced on other weight reduction programs. The diet should only be undertaken with the guidance of a physician, who will prescribe vitamins and minerals and evaluate other individual factors.

So What's Wrong With Pasta?

The answer to this question is long and complex. For those who are not insulin resistant, the reply is probably nothing, so long as they remember that carbohydrates do have calories, and that a low-fat diet is not a license to eat as many sugars and starches as desired. For those who are insulin resistant, however, too much pasta and other carbohydrates, sets in motion a chain of events that may begin with weight gain and then eventually lead to serious heart disease.

Exercise Can Help

Exercise is also important for the person who is insulin resistant. The lipid abnormalities that are typical for the syndrome often include low HDL levels and high triglycerides, conditions that accelerate the development of coronary artery disease even if total cholesterol is low, as is often the case among the insulin resistant. Not only does exercise help raise HDL levels and lower triglycerides, it will help lower the high blood pressure that is part of the syndrome.

Chapter Ten

The Diet

I have always hesitated to hand out diets to people that I don't see in my office. I prefer to individualize an eating program for each person, taking into account his or her health and lifestyle. Along with an individualized eating program, my patients also get an exercise regimen, metabolically enhancing nutrients, and detoxification. Due to popular demand, however, I have devised this one-month insulin-regulating weight loss program that is safe and effective for almost everyone without medical supervision. (The exceptions are people with osteoporosis and kidney and liver disease.)

This is not a fad diet or a quick fix; it requires a commitment from you. When you first look over the eating program, you may think it is too restrictive and that you could never stick to it. But try it. My patients are astonished when they discover how easy it is. If you have only a few pounds to lose, one month on this program may be all you need. If you have a great deal of weight to lose, this diet should be an inspiration, because it will demonstrate conclusively that you can do it if you have the right weight-loss program, and you will be motivated to continue beyond one month. Here then is the diet. Good luck!

The Insulin-Regulating Diet

Breakfast:
Breakfast can be skipped routinely or intermittently. Or, you may have:
- Omelet (two eggs, egg whites only, or egg substitute) with vegetables (peppers, onions, mushrooms) and, if desired, one ounce ham and cheese.
- Two eggs any style. If desired, add two slices of Canadian bacon or two slices soy cheese, or three ounces smoked salmon or other fish or grilled chicken. Or, have any one of these items without the eggs.

Lunch:
- Large salad with olive oil and vinegar. Salad may consist of any of the following: lettuce, watercress, arugula, endive, radishes, spinach, and cucumber.
- Three to five ounces of fish, chicken, or turkey.

Dinner:
- Large salad with oil and vinegar.
- Raw, steamed, or roasted vegetables (cabbage, zucchini, eggplant, leeks, shallots, mushrooms, broccoli, cauliflower, peppers, spinach, fennel, celery, asparagus, string beans, brussel sprouts, or Swiss chard.)
- Three to five ounces fish, chicken or turkey.
- Once a week you may have three to five ounces lean red meat. For very active individuals, the protein portion may be increased.

Between-Meal Snacks:
- One apple per day.
- Three large celery stalks or carrot sticks.
- Two to three ounces tuna fish or grilled chicken.
- Two slices soy cheese or low-fat cheese.

Beverages:
- Water, mineral water, seltzer, unsweetened coffee (black only), or tea.

Vitamin Supplements:
A number of formulations, available from the Wellness Centers, markedly increase the effectiveness of this diet. They are:
- **Carbo Control**: This formula controls insulin and glucose levels, enhances the metabolism, and curbs the appetite.
- A high potency multiple vitamin, such as *Dr. V's Multi-Vite*.
- **DetoxFiber**: This formulation will assist in weight loss by improving intestinal health and removing yeast.
- **Essential Oils**: To improve hormonal and cellular function we recommend replacement with a blend of essential oils.

In addition, every day you should:
- Be sure to drink ten glasses of purified water.
- Take a brisk hour-long walk and work out with weights for an hour.
- Pray or meditate for an hour.
- Record food and beverage intake.
- If you get hungry, drink a glass of water.
- This is a one-month program and should not be used beyond that time unless you consult with us at the Wellness Centers.

INDEX

A

Abiomed, 56
acarbose, 41
ACE inhibitor, 35, 36, 38, 63, 66
acetyicholine, 25
acute myocardial infarction, 45, 64, 3
adult onset diabetes, 128
aging, 24, 25, 65, 83, 91, 94, 100, 101, 105, 108, 130
aging process, 65, 105
AIDS, 94
Alan Ahlschier, 107
alcohol, 21, 53, 61, 62, 76, 116, 118, 119
Altace, 36, 53, 63
American Academy of Anti-Aging Medicine, 106, 109
American College of Cardiology, 3, 45, 46, 62
American Diabetes Association, 97
American Heart Association, 24, 27, 33, 38, 42, 46, 53, 62, 98, 111, 115, 138, 145
American Heart Journal, 64, 3
amino acid, 93, 105, 107, 118, 122
anemia, 96, 123
anencephaly, 93
angina, 34, 37, 39, 45, 47, 52, 89, 112, 118, 134
angiogram, 54
angioplasty, 16, 34, 39, 45, 46, 47, 48, 50, 52, 93
angiotensin-converting emzyme, 35
anticoagulant, 36, 38, 96
aorta, 52, 66
appetite suppressants, 123
argenine, 66
arrhythmia, 51, 66, 117
arrthymias, 97
arthritis, 18, 83, 99, 101, 143
aspirin, 31, 36, 37, 38, 42, 59, 79
atherogenic, 141
atherosclerosis, 5, 16, 17, 22, 24, 47, 50, 112, 127, 128, 132, 135
athletes, 24, 25, 89, 95, 99

Atkins, Robert, 140
Atlantic C-PORT study, 47

B-C

balloon, 16, 45, 48
Barry Sears, 132, 140
Baycol, 31, 32
Bayer, 31
beta radiation, 49
biotin, 120
birth defects, 93
blood clots, 24, 37, 61, 97, 112, 117
blood sugar, 19, 40, 41, 97, 99, 112, 119, 120, 123, 129, 132, 141, 143, 148
Bonnie Liebman, 132
borage oil, 112, 116, 122
brachytherapy, 48, 49
British Medical Journal, 102, 3
bypass surgery, 16, 39, 42, 43, 48, 52, 53, 54, 55, 57, 93, 98
calcium, 87, 88, 97, 103, 104, 117
cancer, 13, 27, 37, 67, 77, 87, 89, 90, 92, 93, 94, 101, 106, 110, 117
candida, 130, 138, 147
carbhydrate addiction, 125, 135, 136, 137
Carbo-Control, 124
Carbohydrate Addict's Lifespan Program, 135, 3
Carbohydrate-Addicted Kids, 144, 3
Cardura, 128
carnathene, 19
carnitine, 88, 89, 99, 122
carotid artery, 127
carotinoids, 89, 90
cataracts, 101
catheterization, 46
cath-lab, 47
central obesity, 126
cerebral aneurysm, 37
Cheney, 9, 47, 49, 50, 51
chest pain, 17, 54, 64, 65, 130, 3
chitosan, 122
cholesterol, 17, 18, 19, 20, 21, 22, 23, 25, 27, 28, 29, 31, 32, 33, 37, 42, 58, 59, 61, 65, 74, 77, 78, 83, 88, 90, 91

glucose intolerance, 97, 120, 121, 126, 129, 131, 132, 133, 138
glucose tolerance, 19, 119, 120, 126, 127, 131
Glucosol, 124
growth hormone, 105, 106, 107, 108, 109, 110, 122, 123, 147
gugulipids, 113

H

Harvard, 4, 36, 37, 93
HDL, 19, 20, 21, 22, 23, 32, 61, 65, 83, 88, 90, 98, 99, 101, 111, 112, 114, 127, 131, 135, 149
health education, 3, 13, 14, 15, 27, 87, 110
Health for Life, 128, 129, 139, 3
healthy heart plan, 17
heart failure, 25, 54, 57, 61, 62, 63, 88, 106, 108
Heart Outcomes Prevention Evaluation, 35
heart-lung machine, 54, 55
Heller, Rachael, 135, 137
Heller, Richard 128, 144
hemorrhoids, 95
HGH, 10, 105, 106, 107, 108, 109, 110, 123, 3, 5
high blood pressure, 18, 19, 28, 37, 42, 63, 65, 66, 79, 92, 95, 97, 110, 111, 114, 115, 116, 120, 125, 127, 129, 131, 133, 135, 136, 138, 141, 143, 148, 149
HMO, 17
Holter monitor, 50
homeostasis, 26
homocysteine, 17, 29, 93
Honolulu Heart Program, 24, 3
HOPE Trials, 35
Howard, George, 126
Human Growth Hormone, 10, 105, 106, 4
hydrogenated oil, 74
hyperinsulinemia, 128, 130, 135
hypertension, 7, 16, 17, 18, 23, 37, 38, 39, 53, 59, 63, 64, 83, 87, 95, 114, 115, 116, 118, 126, 127, 128, 131, 135, 146

I-L

ICD, 51, 52
IGF-1, 109
indulin resistance, 7, 19, 23, 72, 73, 83, 97, 112, 120, 121, 124, 125, 126, 127, 128, 131, 133, 134, 135, 145, 147, 148, 149
insulin, 7, 18, 19, 23, 40, 41, 72, 73, 83, 92, 97, 109, 110, 111, 112, 115, 118, 119, 120, 121, 123, 124, 125, 126, 127, 128, 129, 130, 131, 133, 134, 135, 136, 137, 138, 139, 140, 143, 145, 147, 148, 149, 152
Insulin Growth Factor, 109
insuln regulators, 123
Internet, 15, 16, 27, 56, 57
intestinal dysbiosis, 130
iron, 38, 95, 96
irradiated stents, 49
Johnson & Johnson, 48
Journal of the American Medical Association, 31, 46, 3
Keshan disease, 101
ketosis, 141
kidney disease, 36, 39, 89
kidney stomes, 97
Klatz, Ronald, 106
Korean War Heart Study, 16
laser, 45
L-carnitine, 88, 112, 118, 122
LDL, 17, 19, 20, 21, 22, 23, 25, 32, 33, 59, 98, 99, 101, 112, 113, 114, 126, 131, 143, 145
lecithin, 91
lipid abnormalities, 126, 127, 131, 149
lipid disorders, 33, 126, 127
lipid profile, 20, 22, 88, 97, 98, 101, 128
Lipitor, 31, 34, 53, 59
lipoic acid, 18, 120, 147
liver dease, 37, 41, 62, 89, 150
L-tyrosine, 122

M

ma huang, 122
macular degeneration, 90

magnesium, 19, 96, 97, 112, 116, 117, 123

mammogram, 34

Maria Santoro, 1, 2, 5, 8, 10, 61, 69, 141, 146, 148

Masssachusetts General Hospital, 42

McMaster University, 35

Mediterranean-type diet, 134

Medscape, 54, 58

melatonin, 105, 106

memory, 55, 90, 91, 92, 100, 105, 108

menstruation, 95

Merck, 34

metabolic fitness, 18, 138, 143, 146

metabolic syndrome, 19, 23, 149

metabolism, 23, 83, 90, 91, 105, 120, 122, 123, 129, 148, 152

Mevacor, 31, 34

migraine headache, 97

monounsaturated fats, 134

monounsaturated oils, 20

MSG, 82

myogenisis, 49

N-P

National Academy of Sciences, 102

National Cholesterol Education Program, 19, 20, 21, 22, 23, 33, 149

National Institute of Mental Health, 100

National Institutes of Health, 21, 22, 23, 115

NCEP, 20, 22, 23

neurotransmitters, 87, 91, 100

New Cholesterol Guidelines, 9, 21, 113

New Diet Revolution, 141, 3

New England Jourrnal of Medicne, 36, 103, 106, 108, 115, 144, 145, 4

New York Medical College, 55

New York Times, 31

niacin, 19, 21, 111

nitric oxide, 24, 25

noncardiac chest pain, 54

noncompliance, 42, 58

Nutrition Board, 103

nutritional supplements, 7, 17, 114, 153

nuts, 20, 97, 117

omega-3, 97, 98, 117

Omega-3, 60, 97, 98

Orlistat, 142

Ornish, Dean, 67

oxidative damage, 101

pacemaker, 52

painkillers, 37

panathene, 19

pancreas, 40, 41, 105, 128

pantothenic acid, 99

parasites, 147

pasta, 77, 125, 129, 130, 132, 134, 138, 139, 148, 149

PCI, 45, 46

Pediatrics, 144, 3

peptic ulcer, 95

percutaneous coronary intervention, 45

peripheral vascular disease, 88, 89, 97, 134

PET scan, 16

phentermine, 142

phospholipid, 100

Physician Health Study, 36

pineal gland, 106

pituitary gland, 105, 107

pizza, 68, 70, 75, 140

placebos, 35

plant phytosterols, 113

plaque, 5, 15, 45, 96, 97, 98, 108, 127, 129

platelet, 90, 98, 101

platelet aggregation, 90, 101

Policosonol, 114

potassium, 79, 80, 116, 117

Prandin, 41

Pravachol, 31

Precose, 41

prediabetic, 19, 121, 148

pre-diabetic, 131, 135

pregnenolone, 92

progesterone, 105, 107, 147

prostate cancer, 67, 90, 101

Protein Power, 132, 3

Prozac, 102

Proud, Geoff, 5

PSA, 67

psoriasis, 101

pulmonary disease, 89

pyridoxal 5 phosphate, 124

pyruvate/DHA, 147

pyruvic acid, 122

Bibliography

-Abramson, Jerome, L., et al. "Moderate Alcohol Consumption and Risk of Heart Failure Among Older Persons," *JAMA*, April 18, 2001.

-Atkins, Dr. Robert C., *Dr. Atkins' New Diet Revolution,* William Morrow & Co, 2001.

-Aversano, T. et al., "Percutaneous Coronary Intervention for Myocardial Infarction in Patients Presenting to Hospitals Without On-site Cardiac Surgery," *Journal of the American Medical Association,* April 17, 2002.

-"Beyond Cholesterol: New Uses for Statins," *American Medical News*, June 18, 2001, www.amednews.com.

-Cook, Nancy R., et al., "Self-Selected Post-trial Aspirin Use and Subsequent Cardiovascular Disease and Mortality in the Physicians' Health Study," *Archives of Internal Medicine,* April 10, 2000.

-Eades, Michael and Mary, *Protein Power,* Bantam Books, 1996.

-Fletcher, Anne M., *Thin for Life,* Harper Collins 1994.

-Hakim, A.A., et al., "Effects of walking on coronary heart disease in elderly men: the Honolulu Heart Program." Circulation, vol. 100 (1999)* http.//circ.ahajournals.org/search.dtl.

-Heller, Rachael and Richard, *The Carbohydrate Addict's Healthy for Life,* Dutton Plume, 1996.

-Heller, Rachael and Richard, *Carbohydrate-Addicted Kids,* Paperback Harper Trade, 1998.

-Heller, Rachael and Richard, *The Carbohydrate Addict's Lifespan Program,* Dutton Plume, 1996.

-Herlitz, Johan, et al., "Important factors for the 10-year mortality rate in patients with acute chest pain or other symptoms consistent with acute myocardial infarction with particular emphasis on the influence of age," *American Heart Journal,* October 2001.

-Katz, Dr. Ronald, *Grow Young with HGH,* HarperCollins Publishers, 1997.

-Kimmel, Stephen E., et al., "Effects of Coronary Stents on Cardiovascular Outcomes in Broad-Based Clinical Practice," *Archives of Internal Medicine,* September 25, 2000.

-LaRosa, John C., et al., "Effect of Statins on Risk of Coronary Diseases: A Meta-analysis of Randomized Controlled Trials," *Journal of the American Medical Association*, Vol. 282, December 22, 1999.

-Linde, K., et al. "St. John's wort for depression—an overview and meta-analysis of randomized clinical trials," *British Medical Journal,* August 3, 1996.

-Muñoz, Kathyrn A., et al., "Food Intakes of US Children and Adolescents Compared With Recommendations," *Pediatrics*, September 1997.

-Ornish, Dean, M.D., *Love and Survival: Eight Pathways to Intimacy and Health ,* HarperPerennial, NY, 1998.

-Pfisterer, M.E., "The TIME Study," *XX III Annual Congress Stockholm 2001,* European Society of Cardiology.

-Rocchini, A.P., "Childhood Obesity and a Diabetes Epidemic," *New England Journal of Medicine,* March 14, 2002.

-Rosenthal, N., "High Hopes for the Heart," (Editorial), *New England Journal of Medicine,* June 7, 2001.

-Rudman, D., et al., "Effects of Human Growth Hormone," *New England Journal of Medicine,* July 5,1990.

-Sears, Dr. Barry, *The Zone: A Dietary Roadmap,* Harper Collins, 1995.

-Secades, J.J., Frontera, G., "CDP-choline: Pharmaceutical and clinical review," *Methods and Findings in Experimental Clinical Pharmacology,* vol. 17 (1995).

-Sotile, Wayne, Ph.D., *Heart Illness and Intimacy,* Books on Demand, 1992.

-Taddei, Stefano, et al., "Physical Activity Prevents Age-Related Impairment in Nitric Oxide Availability in Elderly Athletes," Circulation vol. 101 (2000) http.//circ.ahajournals.org/search.dtl.

-Thomas, M.K., et al., "Hypovitaminosis D in medical inpatients," *New England Journal of Medicine*, March 19, 1998.

-Warner, Jennifer, "Brain May Suffer Long After Heart Bypass," *WebMD Medical News,* July 15, 2002.

-Weintraub, William S., "Commentary," *Journal of Invasive Cardiology*, November, 2000.

Other Books by Safe Goods

All-Natural High Performance Diet	$ 7.95US $11.95CA
The Sugar Addict's Diet	$12.95US $19.95CA
Nutritional Leverage for Great Golf	$ 9.95US $14.95CA
Feeling Younger with Homeopathic HGH	$ 7.95US $11.95CA
The Natural Prostate Cure	$ 6.95 US $10.95 CA
Natural Born Fatburners	$14.95US $22.95CA
Lower Cholesterol without Drugs	$ 6.95US $10.95CA
Macrobiotics for Americans	$ 7.95 US $11.95 CA
Cancer Disarmed	$ 4.95 US $ 6.95 CA

For a complete listing of books visit our website
www.safegoodspub.com
or call for a free catalog (888) 628-8731
order line: (888) NATURE-1